PRAISE FOR *Gracefully Insane*:

"[Beam] elicits fascinating stories from both residents and staff . . . [and] . . . has nicely traced the history of this institution and its inhabitants."

Entertainment Weekly

"Beam tells good stories and with an appropriate tone—intrigued and respectful, but not pious."

Washington Post

"A brilliant blend of substance, story, and commentary, *Gracefully Insane* is at once an academic exploration of an institution and an insightful glimpse inside troubled lives."

Boston Magazine

"A lucid, compelling social and cultural history of a segment of American life that is worthy of both James brothers: Henry's story-telling gifts and his discerning eye for class and its psychological consequences, and William's knowing medical awareness. . . . A major narrative achievement."

Robert Coles

"[A] fascinating, gossipy social history . . . More than a history of a psychiatric institution, the book offers an unusual glimpse of a celebrated American estate: the Boston aristocracy . . . "

Publishers Weekly

"An engaging history of the psychiatric treatment of the American socioeconomic elite since the early 19th century."

Barron's Financial Review

"Alex Beam packs the whole history of psychiatry into the biography of a single institution that for nearly 200 years has offered refuge to some of America's most talented thinkers and artists. . . . A gracious, gossipy, well-informed, page-turner of a book, a pleasure to read."

Diane Middlebrook

"An admirable institutional history, and more so, a captivating social history, for what makes McLean distinctive, its style and sensibility, is part and parcel of what Boston, as a cultural instance, represents."

Kirkus Reviews

"Often fascinating . . . , the book weaves together the compelling history of McLean and those who came seeking its refuge."

Book Magazine

"Combines the history of McLean Hospital with reflections on the history of psychiatry. The result is a wonderful book for psychologists, psychiatrists, and history buffs—and for anyone interested in mental health."

Steven Pinker

"An oddly entertaining narrative that reads easily and supplies fascinating details about business, pop music, and literary figures."

Library Journal

Gracefully Insane

ALSO BY ALEX BEAM

Fellow Travelers
The Americans Are Coming!

Gracefully INSANE

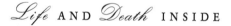 *Life* AND *Death* INSIDE

AMERICA'S PREMIER MENTAL HOSPITAL

ALEX BEAM

PublicAffairs
New York

Book design by Jane Raese

Library of Congress Cataloging-in-Publication Data
Beam, Alex.
Gracefully insane : life and death inside America's premier mental hospital /
by Alex Beam. – 1st ed.
p. cm.
Includes index.
ISBN 1-58648-161-4 / (pbk.)
1. McLean Hospital–History. I. Title.
RC445.M4 B442 2001
362.2'1'097444–dc21
2001048339

To my mother and father

Contents

. . . (This is the house for the "mentally ill.")

What use is my sense of humor?
I grin at Stanley, now sunk in his sixties,
once a Harvard all-American fullback
(if such were possible!)
still hoarding the build of a boy in his twenties,
as he soaks, a ramrod
with the muscle of a seal
in his long tub,
vaguely urinous from the Victorian plumbing,
A kingly granite profile in a crimson golf-cap,
worn all day, all night,
he thinks only of his figure
of slimming on sherbet and ginger ale—
more cut off from words than a seal.

This is the way day breaks in Bowditch Hall at McLean's;
the hooded night lights bring out "Bobbie,"
Porcellian '29
a replica of Louis XVI
without the wig—
redolent and roly-poly as a sperm whale,

as he swashbuckles about in his birthday suit
and horses at chairs.

These victorious figures of bravado ossified young.
In between the limits of day,
hours and hours go by under the crew haircuts
and slightly too little nonsensical bachelor twinkle
of the Roman Catholic attendants.
(There are no Mayflower
screwballs in the Catholic Church.)

After a hearty New England breakfast,
I weigh two hundred pounds
this morning. Cock of the walk,
I strut in my turtle-necked French sailor's jersey
before the metal shaving mirrors,
and see the shaky future grow familiar
in the pinched, indigenous faces
of these thoroughbred mental cases,
twice my age and half my weight.
We are all old-timers,
each of us holds a locked razor.

from "Waking in the Blue," by Robert Lowell

1

A Visit to the Museum
of the Cures

Everyone makes the same comment: It doesn't look like a mental hospital. The carefully landscaped grounds, dotted with four- and five-story Tudor mansions and red brick dormitories, could belong to a prosperous New England prep school or perhaps a small, well-endowed college tucked away in the Boston suburbs. There are no fences, no guards, no locked gates. Over time, of course, you see the signs. Iron grilles surround the staircases inside the few remaining locked wards. On some halls, the nurses' stations are enclosed in thick Plexiglas. The washroom mirrors are polished metal, not glass. But on first acquaintance, the only indication that you have entered one of America's oldest and most prestigious mental hospitals is a large sign jutting into Mill Street: McLean Hospital.

Although I had already interviewed several doctors in their offices, I took my first formal tour of the campus on a sunny, early-summer Saturday in 1998. McLean was hosting an orientation meeting for its neighbors in the well-to-do town of Belmont, Massachusetts. Our group of twenty could just as well have been bird watchers out for a jaunt. In fact, as we strode along the sculptured walkways cut through the scrubby New England forest, several men and women revealed themselves to be Audubon Society members, who instantly recognized the hospital's dense stands of oak and elm forests as nesting grounds for red-tailed hawk and horned and screech owls. There were two "soccer moms" in our group, real soccer moms, it turns out–they *played* soccer. Everyone was wearing sensible clothing for our tour of what was once America's premier insane asylum.

McLean was showing off its 240-acre campus to promote its new Hospital Re-Use Master Plan. Starting in the 1980s, neither private insurers nor government programs like Medicare and Medicaid were willing to finance the lengthy stays and staff-intensive therapy that had been McLean's specialty for almost two centuries. Whereas once well-heeled patients had checked in for months' if not years' worth of expensive, residential therapy, the standard admission was now the "five-day": time enough for a quick psychiatric diagnosis, stabilization on drugs, and release "into the community," meaning to a halfway house or, in the most hopeful scenario, back to one's family. By the early 1990s, McLean was losing millions of dollars a year. It came within a hair's breadth of being closed down. The hospital was foundering like a luxury ocean liner competing in the age of jet travel.

To save McLean, the businessmen who sat on the board of trustees opted to "restructure" the hospital. McLean had already shrunk dramatically; in the late 1990s, staffers were preparing just 100 beds a night, compared with 340 during most of the twentieth century. Entire buildings had already been closed. "It occurred to us that we had about 250 acres and 800,000 square feet of building space, and given the profile of the way we were delivering the medicine, we probably needed only 50 acres and 300,000 square feet," Charles Baker, a former chairman of the board, explained to me. The eventual Master Plan called for selling off about half the asylum's acreage and keeping an inner core of fifty acres for patient treatment and research labs. The rest would be given to the town as public open space. The idea was to raise $40 million, erase the hospital's outstanding debt, and rescue McLean.

The tours eventually had the desired impact; after years of town-gown bickering, Belmont finally voted to allow McLean to de-accession its real estate treasures in 1999. McLean had signed a deal to turn twelve acres of scrub forest on its southern perimeter into a mirror-windowed, 300,000-square-foot biomedical research park of the kind to be seen on the outskirts of Princeton, Atlanta, Seattle, or pretty much any white-collar, city-suburb in America. Twenty-six acres along busy Mill Street will be developed for town houses, to be priced between $600,000 and $650,000. At a separate briefing, an official of the Northland Development Corporation showed us how the new homes would be painted in earth colors, surrounded by trees, and kept low to the ground so as not to change the profile of the west-facing wooded hill. He briefly addressed the potential challenge of selling expensive homes abutting the grounds of an insane asylum, but he hoped it would not be a problem.

Down the hill from the town houses, McLean has convinced the American Retirement Corporation to build a 352-unit "eldercare center," an upscale retirement home. Other plots have been earmarked to placate various constituencies that hold McLean's fate in their hands. The 130 acres of open space, some of it abutting an Audubon Society sanctuary, should quiet Belmont's vocal environmentalists. The hospital will donate one and a half acres to expand—and silence—a neighboring housing development for the elderly. A private school on the hospital's northern border will get land for a new soccer field. And the town fathers of Belmont will be rewarded with twenty acres for their long-standing pet project, a cemetery expansion.

Throughout the process, McLean, a teaching hospital of Harvard University, has behaved with perfect decorum. I attended a citizens' meeting where an abutter who opposed the Master Plan objected to the "quick fix" cemetery expansion, which, he complained, would serve Belmont's needs for only the next seventy-five years. A development staffer working with the hospital replied, "We'll show you a picture of a forest cemetery in Sweden," invoking the Scandinavian penchant for tasteful, appropriately scaled development, even for cemeteries. At a Belmont Conservation Commission meeting, a small group of environmentalists demanded special consideration for a tiny brook flowing down the southern slope of the site of the proposed office park development, a stream that eventually reaches the Mystic River. The McLean lawyers huddled briefly and then agreed not to disturb any land within one hundred feet of the running water.

Although it still functions as a mental hospital, McLean is also a living museum. It is a museum of the grand Boston culture that was, for a century or more, synonymous with American culture. The names of the older houses we encounter on our tour—Appleton, Bowditch, Codman, Higginson—are the names of the roving ship captains who enriched and ennobled the Boston of the 1800s. Henry Lee Higginson was the man who founded the Boston Symphony Orchestra and later became an activist member of Harvard's governing corporation. Higginson is still remembered for a Harvard fund-raising letter that ended with this line: "Educate, and save ourselves and our families and our money from mobs!" William Appleton, a major nineteenth-century donor, was a typical Yankee trader; he freely admitted in his posthumously published diary that "my mind is very much bent on making money." He referred to his marriage as "a Matrimonial Speculation, the whole result of which is not ascertained." In addition to giving buildings, Appleton also created a special fund in the 1830s to help defray treatment costs of "desirable" patients for whom the initial $2.50-a-week cost was too steep.

Bowditch Hall is named for Nathaniel Ingersoll Bowditch, another great name from the sea. A sailor-mathematician, Bowditch's subtle improvements on celestial navigation allowed the Boston clipper captains, like John Codman and his heirs, to beat their competitors to Japan. More than one hundred years after its publication, his *Practical Navigator* remained the standard treatise in its field. When Bowditch died in 1838, captains of American, English, and Russian vessels in the Russian port of Kronstadt flew their flags at half-mast, and the cadets at Annapolis wore badges of mourning.

A century and a half later a young Boston writer and explorer, Rob Perkins, wrote a memoir about being a patient on Bowditch Hall:

> Navigation is the art of going from what you know to what you don't know. The hall is named after Nathaniel Bowditch, another rigid man, the father of navigation. For centuries ships depended on his system. They went around the world on it, across oceans. For all I know, NASA sends up their rockets with his knowledge. It's all math and rational. There are many ways to navigate, but even knowing how doesn't necessarily keep you off the rocks. The man went nuts. His family locked him up in McLean Hospital. Later, they named the maximum security hall after him. There is a statue of him in Mount Auburn Cemetery holding a globe and a sextant in his lap. There is also a waiting list to get into both places, Bowditch and Mount Auburn Cemetery.

Bowditch also was the stomping ground of Robert Lowell, the blue-blood poet who immortalized the locked men's ward in a famous poem, "Waking in the Blue" ("This is the way day breaks at Bowditch Hall at McLean's"). Lowell published his second volume of poems while at McLean. He even corresponded with

Jacqueline Kennedy and Ezra Pound from the hospital. In his manic phases, Lowell held court at Bowditch. A visitor once saw him haranguing a small crowd of patients and staff while sitting on the bed of a young man named John Forbes Nash, who had been involuntarily committed from the Massachusetts Institute of Technology (MIT) in 1959. Lowell was a celebrity; when he showed up at McLean, "it was like seeing Princess Diana," one staffer remembers. But no one knew who Nash was or that he had already finished the research in game theory that would later win him a Nobel Prize. Two future Pulitzer Prizes (Lowell's) and a future Nobel in one room. An ordinary day on the wards at McLean.

I had never seen Appleton, the laid-back coed ward for the 1960s generation, nor Codman before. Codman, now closed, was once the women's geriatric ward. Psychiatrist Robert Coles remembers the "crazy ladies of Codman," who staged elaborate tea parties on silver service for him and other young residents in the late 1950s.

Wheeling back toward the Bowl, a perfect, concave expanse of grass where psychiatrists and patients used to play golf together, we pass South Belknap, originally the Belknap House for Women. Belknap is the "Belsize" of Sylvia Plath's novel, *The Bell Jar*. When the fictional Esther Greenwood "moves 'up' to Belsize," she knows she is getting better. Plath observed, but did not celebrate, her twenty-first birthday at McLean and was elected to the Phi Beta Kappa Society while on the wards. Belknap was also a temporary home for Susanna Kaysen, the daughter of President John F. Kennedy's deputy national security adviser; she later wrote a best-selling memoir of her stay at McLean, *Girl, Interrupted*. One of Kaysen's ward mates was Kate Taylor, the daughter of the dean of the University of North Carolina Medical School. One day in 1968, Kate showed the other girls on her ward a test pressing of a record called simply *James Taylor*, which was soon to become the number-one-selling album in the country. One of the songs, "Knockin' 'Round the Zoo," was about McLean. Smiling, wagging his head mournfully before youthful audiences all over the country, Kate's brother James would joke about his "degree" from McLean. Kate would have her own successful recording career. Her brother Livingston, who also punched his ticket at McLean, wrote a song that mentioned his favorite McLean doctor.

But even in the field of music, the Taylors were not McLean's most distinguished "graduates." That accolade would go to Ray Charles, who overlapped with Taylor at McLean in the mid-1960s. Following Charles's arrest at Logan Airport for possession of heroin, a broad-minded federal judge allowed the singer to kick the habit at McLean instead of rotting away in jail. Charles turned out to be a satisfied customer and a repeat visitor. In his autobiography, he reminisces about playing the piano on a minimum-security ward and "getting next to" the McLean nurses. Clay Jackson, a legendary musician from the heyday of Cambridge's Club 47—Joan Baez's first concert venue*—and two of Van Morrison's brilliant sidemen also passed through McLean. They could have had a hell of a band.

As our tour inspects the proposed location for the biomedical office complex, I catch my first view of East House, a three-story Jacobean revival mansion originally designed to shelter thirty women patients in individual suites. After World War II, it became the women's maximum-security ward. A disturbing rash of suicides erupted at East House in 1960 and spread across the campus. I have a mimeographed collection of poems called "Behind the Screen: Poems from the Female Maximum Security Hall" written by three East House patients in 1969. About half the poems concern suicide.

Descending from Bowditch, we stroll through a perfectly arrayed orchard and catch a glimpse of the huge barn, once the cen-

---

*I found the following entry in the August 15, 1960, edition of the patient-edited newsletter, "Around and About McLean": "There's a real treat in store for us next Tuesday night at the P.A.A. [Patient Activities Association] get-together at 7:30. Miss Joan Baez will entertain, singing ballads and accompanying herself on the guitar. This will be a return engagement for Miss Baez, who has played twice recently at Codman and once before at P.A.A."

terpiece of a working farm that provided the hospital with its own milk, eggs, and produce up until 1942. With the onset of World War II, the livestock had to be killed to provide meat for GI rations. A few riding horses, available for patients and staff, were kept in the barn until the 1960s. One of the hospital executives leading our tour marvels that McLean was a self-sufficient community just fifty years earlier. It had its own operating rooms, tennis courts, music, theater and movie shows, and of course its own hair salon and barber. There was even a small chapel, built by the Eliots with stained-glass windows donated by other First Families—the Beebes, Noyes, Kidders, and Shaws. Back then, the entire staff—the Harvard Medical School–trained doctors, the immigrant nurses, and even the janitors—lived on campus. Not so long ago, the only time McLean employees telephoned to the town of Belmont was to summon the coroner to package up the occasional corpse.

At odd moments during our walk, huge, spreading, seventy-foot-tall copper beeches heave into view. The staffers accompanying us seem well briefed; they know the fate of each of these towering, golden-brown giants. "This one is slated for preservation. . . . This one over here? No, this is where the parking lot will be." Trees are a very big deal at McLean. The developers working on each of the commercial parcels had to inventory every tree more than two feet tall and have practically apologized personally each time a "signature tree" has been cut down or replanted. Indeed, a forester employed by Northland reminded a McLean gathering I attended that New England is now far more wooded than it was 150 years ago, when most of the land had been cleared for agriculture.

Virtually every doctor more than sixty years old has a copy of the hand-drawn poster "The Trees of McLean" hanging on his or her office wall. Created by two patients with the help of a specialist from Harvard's Arnold Arboretum in 1966, it is a precise map of each important tree on the McLean grounds. One of the creators, Stewart Sanders, went on to become a prominent naturalist in the Boston area. In later years, he performed the Audubon Society Christmas bird count on the McLean grounds and even drafted maps of fox habitats and woodcock flight patterns that included some of the hospital territory. "I wanted to control people's actions in the future," Sanders told me. "I was showing that this was where the trees were, this was where the foxes were so that they wouldn't be disturbed." Now in his sixties, Sanders is a studious yet emotional defender of open space in the Boston area. He was one of the men who won the hundred-foot setback for the threatened brook at the Conservation Commission hearing. "I gave an emotional plea that when the people of Massachusetts enacted the Rivers Protection Act, they meant to include brooks, because they understood that brooks become rivers. It's very nice that they have fountains at the Burlington Mall, but my heart needs a brook."

It is impossible not to be transported by the beauty of McLean. "We are very proud of our hospital. It is very attractive and looks more like a college campus than a mental hospital," the Babbitty World War II-era director Franklin Wood once boasted. (Wood was an occasional source of unintended humor. Rejecting a suggestion by patients that he erect signs to guide them around the grounds, he said, "If you don't know where you are, then you're in the right place." Writing in the hospital's annual report, he contributed this gem: "It is not healthy to be depressed.") Four-fifths of the grounds are just that: grounds, not buildings. This is the patch of rolling, rocky New England woodland that the great landscape designer Frederick Law Olmsted chose for McLean in the late nineteenth century. Olmsted knew what he wanted: a setting that would allow every patient's window to face south and that would have enough space so that the men's buildings would not look in on the women's wards. He foresaw that patients should be segregated according to the acuity of their illnesses. He surveyed two other sites but favored "the wooded land of Belmont, judiciously thinned to groups and glades, opened by walks of long curves, and easy slope." It would provide, he wrote to the hospital

trustees, "more incitements to tranquilizing and recreative volun-
tary exercise for convalescent and harmless monomaniac patients"
than would rival parcels in Arlington and Waltham. Twenty-five
years later, Olmsted, debilitated by a series of brain hemorrhages,
found himself living in McLean's Hope Cottage, a single-patient
home perched on a ridge above a terraced hillside garden. He had
lost many of his faculties but not his sense of orientation. Ever the
landscape connoisseur, Olmsted noticed that the buildings were
not as tightly grouped as he had suggested in an 1875 sketch for
the trustees. Moreover, they now faced the beautiful western sun-
set and not the southern horizon, as he had recommended. Surveying the setting, he exclaimed: "They didn't follow my plan,
confound them!"

McLean Hospital is not just a cultural museum. It is also a museum
of the many therapies advanced over more than two hundred
years to relieve mental illness. In large part, the story of McLean is
the story of an idea that originated in Europe at the end of the
eighteenth century. The idea was that a relaxed life in a pastoral
setting would go a long way toward alleviating the suffering of the
mentally ill.

The theory's most famous champion was Philippe Pinel, an en-
lightened French doctor to whom the Revolutionary government
had handed the keys of Paris's most notorious hellhole, the Bicetre Asylum, in 1792. Pinel was a failed rural practitioner who had
devoted himself to the study of mental illness after a friend suffered a nervous breakdown, fled into a forest, and was devoured
by wolves. "The Bicetre," wrote historian Albert Deutsch, "owned
a questionable distinction: it ranked with the worst asylums in the
world. There the patients, or rather the inmates, were loaded
down with chains and shackled to floors and walls with irons, at
the mercy of cruel attendants armed with whips and the authority

to use them freely." (Terrorizing mental patients, in the hopes of "waking" them from madness, was common all over Europe. One German asylum lowered patients into a dungeon filled with snakes. Even England's King George III was beaten by an attendant during one of his asylum stays.) Pinel's first act, immortalized in a famous painting by Robert Fleury that shows a patient kissing his hand in gratitude, was to strike the chains off fifty-three of the filthy, bedraggled "beasts" that had been remanded to his care. Most of them proved to be quite harmless. Their previously violent behavior had mimicked the violence visited upon them by their keepers. Pinel introduced elementary hygiene, humane living conditions, and occupational therapies as substitutes for the leg irons, whippings, and brutal beatings that were the norm in European and American asylums. The same year in England, a Quaker named William Tuke founded the York Retreat for the mentally disturbed, a manor house so named "to convey the idea of what such an institution should be, namely, a place in which the unhappy might obtain a refuge; a quiet haven in which the shattered bark might find the means of reparation and safety."

The new movement had a name: moral treatment. A New York doctor named T. Romeyn Beck laid out its tenets in 1811:

> This consists in moving patients from their residence to some proper asylum; and for this purpose a calm retreat in the country is to be preferred: for it is found that continuance at home aggravates the diseases, as the improper association of ideas cannot be destroyed. A system of human vigilance is adopted. Coercion by blows, stripes and chains, although sanctioned by the authority of Celsus and Cullen, is now justly laid aside. . . .
>
> Tolerate noisy ejaculations; strictly exclude visitors; let their fears and resentments be soothed without unnecessary opposition; adopt a system of regularity; make them rise, take exercise and food at stated times. . . .
>
> When convalescing, allow limited liberty; introduce entertaining books and conversation, exhilarating music, employment of body in

agricultural pursuits . . . and admit friends under proper restrictions. It will also be proper to forbid [the patients] returning home too soon. By thus acting, the patient will "minister to himself."

Beck's outline could have served as a mission statement for McLean; for its predecessor, the Philadelphia Hospital; for the Bloomingdale Asylum outside New York; for the Hartford Retreat; or for the Menninger Clinic through the first half of the twentieth century. More than a hundred years after Beck wrote, McLean's superintendent George Tuttle had this to say about the hospital "cures" of 1913: "There have been no striking changes during the year in methods of treatment. Emphasis is still laid on the superior advantage of out-of-door exercise, full feeding, and hydrotherapy for its tonic or soothing effect, as against sedative and hypnotic drugs, which practically are never prescribed."

The hydrotherapy treatment that Tuttle mentions likewise dates back to the eighteenth century. Another famous French painting, Jacques-Louis David's *The Death of Marat,* depicts the emaciated revolutionary slumped over in the bath in his home, after being fatally stabbed by Charlotte Corday. You cannot tell by looking at the Bowditch and Wyman buildings that a half-century ago, the basements of these stately halls were given over to hydrotherapy baths just like those in the David painting, with their long tubs and sail-like canvas covers intended to prevent patients from drowning. (Some did anyway.) The so-called Scotch douches, showers in which the patients were surrounded by needle-like jets of water and then hosed down with ice-cold water from chrome-plated fire hoses—"medieval torture instrument[s]," one doctor called them—were dismantled in the 1950s.

Over the years, McLean supplemented the rest cure with the various weapons that appear and disappear in the psychiatric armamentarium. Only a historian, or a doctor past retirement age, would recognize such terms as "total push," "metrazol shock therapy," or the most alluring of the lot, the "continuous sleep cure."

And yet everything that was old becomes new again. Electroshock therapy, now rebranded "electroconvulsive therapy (ECT)," is still prescribed for recurring, stubborn depression.* The days when Dr. Walter Freeman barnstormed the country in his Cortez camper-van, proselytizing for while-you-wait ice-pick lobotomies for patients "sedated" by electroshock, are history. But selective psychosurgery still figures in the mental health portfolio. And imagine my surprise when I read in a 1999 McLean brochure that "Milieu Therapy is Alive and Well," which of course it is. The impetus behind milieu, a 1950s coinage, is almost exactly analogous to Pinel's eighteenth-century intuition that mental patients, like anyone else, might be able to shed some of the stress and pains of their afflictions in the bucolic environment of a suburban hospital.

The idea of a rest cure, supplemented with occupational therapies, physical therapies, or talk therapies, seems natural to us. But it has proved to be an idea that we can no longer afford to believe in. First-class asylum care, characterized by lengthy stays and solicitous medical attention, has not been particularly successful. So-called outcome statistics are notoriously unreliable when judging mental hospitals. A hospital that specializes in the "worried well" will discharge many patients claiming to have recovered. But institutions like McLean, which has always been willing to grapple with schizophrenia and other severe disturbances, will not have a stellar success record. Perhaps one-third of severely disturbed patients improve under hospital care and leave in better shape than they came. Another one-third can be stabilized and show only marginal improvement; this group can be weaned from full-time care. And the rest probably belong in the hospital full-time.

These days, neither individuals nor insurance companies can afford to pay for residential care. A night at McLean now costs al-

---

*McLean's current literature emphasizes that this isn't your grandfather's shock therapy: "Although ECT was introduced in the 1930s, its therapeutic use today is very different from what is portrayed as 'shock treatment' in books and films. ECT, in fact, is a safe, effective procedure provided by highly skilled professionals" and so on and so forth.

most $900. For the past twenty-five years, we have been embarked on a different path for treating the mentally ill. Ever since the emergence of Thorazine, the immobilizing "prescription strait-jacket" introduced into widespread use in the late 1950s, drug ther-apy has supplanted asylum care as the order of the day. "Now they lock you up in a chemical jail," is how James Taylor–who has been drug-free for almost twenty years–describes modern psychia-try. Yet for as much as it has been criticized, the "psychopharma-ceutical revolution" has proved to be cost-effective in many instances. Now, severely disturbed patients can often live in half-way houses or low-security settings. Many drugs successfully treat, or at least ameliorate, conditions such as depression or compul-sive disorders. But the causes and potential cures for schizophre-nia–the "broken mind"–are still largely unknown. "Researchers are still in the dark about schizophrenia," a March 2001 issue of the *Harvard Mental Health Newsletter* admitted. Mental health is the question for which we have yet to learn the answer. This book is, in part, a history of that question, and the many suggested answers.

But it is also a book about people. The last person quoted here is a patient, not a doctor, and a patient embarked, hopefully, on the road to a better life. People ask me why I undertook this proj-ect, and I have a series of responses, depending on their actual level of interest. Because McLean is an interesting place, full of great stories, I say. That ends most conversations. Because it was a challenge, I say to others; such a book has not been written. That satisfies many questioners. But one afternoon at the Iruna, the de-lightfully down-at-the-mouth Spanish café across from Harvard's John F. Kennedy School of Government, Rob Perkins asked me why I had chosen to spend several years of my life researching the hospital. Rob had spent almost two years' hard time as a patient at McLean and had written movingly about his experiences there. I respected him enormously, and I could not buffalo him the way I could everyone else. "Rob, life is impossible," I confessed. "Who can't understand the need for shelter? And who can't sympathize with the people who seek that shelter? And who could fail to be interested in a place that offered that shelter?"

So this is a book about the men and women who needed shelter more than most of us, or who, in some cases, were more honest about their need for protection than we are. And about an institution that provided that shelter, imperfectly, in our imperfect world.

2

By the Best People, for the Best People

Crazy people much more pleasant than I expected.
McLean pharmacist William Folsom, 1825

By the early nineteenth century, the city of Boston was already two hundred years old. The great Yankee trades to Europe, the Caribbean, and the Far East were pouring money into the counting houses of India Wharf and into the vaults of new banks springing up on State Street. Boston, given to calling itself the "Athens of America," was locked in a grand rivalry with Philadelphia and New York and hooked on new construction. The society architect Charles Bulfinch was remaking the face of the city, planting his distinctive, boxy, brick, federalist mansions along Boston's main thoroughfares, culminating in his gold-domed masterwork, the Commonwealth's State House atop Beacon Hill. The city had just built five bridges spanning the Charles River. The first interurban railroad, the Boston and Albany line, was about to begin service. The city fathers trained in 7,700 tons of marble from Quincy quarries to erect the 220-foot-tall Bunker Hill monument, commemorating the famous battle, and imposed upon the doddering Marquis de Lafayette to lay the cornerstone.

And yet Boston lacked a hospital.

New York, Baltimore, Philadelphia, and even Williamsburg, Virginia, had been operating large public hospitals for more than fifty years, all of which accepted mental patients as well as the sick and infirm. But Boston maintained only a quarantine station on nearby Rainsford Island and the public dispensary, which gave outpatient care to the poor. The mad or delirious were either cared for at home, packed off to the (Bulfinch-designed) Almshouse for the destitute, or farmed out to specialized boarding houses. In his book *The Mentally Ill in America,* Albert Deutsch mentions a

Dr. Willard, who, about the beginning of the 19th century, maintained a private establishment for the mentally ill in a little town between Massachusetts and Rhode Island. One of the fundamental tenets in his therapy was to break the patient's will by any means possible. On his premises stood a tank of water, into which a patient, packed into a coffin-like box pierced with holes, was lowered by means of a well-sweep. He was kept under water until the bubbles of air ceased to rise, after which he was taken out, rubbed, and revived—if he had not already passed beyond reviving!

Two physicians from esteemed Boston First Families, James Jackson and John Collins Warren—it was Warren's uncle who urged the Colonials not to fire until they saw the whites of their British enemies' eyes on Bunker Hill—adopted the hospital cause and circulated a petition to the city's Yankee oligarchs in 1810:

Sir—It has appeared very desirable to a number of respectable gentlemen, that a hospital for the reception of lunatics and other sick persons should be established in this town. . . .

The virtuous and industrious are liable to become objects of public charity, in consequence of the diseases of the mind. When those who are unfortunate in this respect are left without proper care, a calamity, which might have been transient, is prolonged through life.

Jackson and Warren, "charter members in a society that had only charter members" as Cleveland Amory called them, reminded the Puritan legatees of their responsibilities:

It is unnecessary to urge the propriety and even the obligation of succoring the poor in sickness. The wealthy inhabitants of the town of Boston always evinced that they consider themselves as "treasurers of God's bounty"; and in Christian countries it must always be considered the first of duties to visit and to heal the sick. . . . It is worthy of the opulent men of this town, and consistent with the general character, to provide an asylum for the insane from every part of the Commonwealth.

The doctors' plea did not fall on deaf ears. But it did fall on the ears of merchant princes who were temporarily short on cash. Thomas Jefferson's foreign trade embargo had ended only the previous year. Moreover, the reason for the embargo—the diplomatic complications of Europe's Napoleonic Wars—had not disappeared. Indeed, things would get worse before they got better. The British blockaded American ports during the War of 1812 and paralyzed Yankee shipping. Jackson and Warren failed to raise the needed funds.

They did, however, obtain a charter from the Commonwealth of Massachusetts and formed a corporation of fifty-five members. Then as now, the trustees of the Massachusetts General Hospital and the Charlestown (later McLean) Asylum hailed from the New

World aristocracy. Former president John Adams moderated the first meeting. Other members included his son, the future president John Quincy Adams, a future vice-president, a future Supreme Court justice, and a future Harvard president. By the end of the war, economic health was restored, and the merged hospital projects moved forward. The asylum, sited on a spit of land overlooking the harbor in Charlestown, opened its doors in 1817, several years before the Massachusetts General Hospital. (At midcentury, this area incorporated itself as Somerville, and McLean was sometimes called the Somerville Asylum.) This was partly because Jackson, Warren, and their supporters raised money for the asylum more quickly than for the hospital and partly because they happened upon a fortuitous real estate deal for McLean.

The ill fortunes of one Joseph Barrell, who had once employed the architect Bulfinch in his counting house, proved to be a boon for the asylum. Barrell, a horticultural enthusiast, had built what some thought to be the most beautiful country home in New England, an eighteen-acre estate adorned with hundreds of ornamental plants and fruit trees imported from Europe. He had embellished the property with stables, dovecotes, greenhouses, a rose-covered summerhouse, fountains, and even exotic fish pools. His terraced gardens swept down to the water. Atop them sat a Bulfinch-designed, three-story, English-style manor house with a southern view over Miller's Creek, a tributary of the Charles, and an eastern exposure to the river's mouth and the harbor.

But Barrell luxuriated in his Charlestown aerie for less than ten years before succumbing to debts and death in 1804. In 1816, the hospital trustees bought the estate for just $15,650, a great bargain compared with the $23,000 they paid just a few months later for the four acres of undeveloped Boston land that was to become the Massachusetts General Hospital. After the purchase of the Barrell estate, Bulfinch added three-story wings to each side of his brick manor house—a men's ward and a women's ward—and the new asylum opened for business.

For several years, McLean was the only mental hospital in Boston, and it attracted a fairly diverse patient population. Still, because the incorporators did not want their new hospital to become "a merely pauper establishment," they successfully resisted the legislature's demand that they admit charity patients for free. Instead, they assessed fees on a sliding scale. Charity cases dependent on municipal support were billed $2.50 a week, to be paid by their town of residence. The administration reserved the right to show preference for donors' families or for patients from towns that had aided the hospital financially. Patients trickled in, which was fine with the administrators, who were learning on the job. Patient Number One, as McLean's official historian Silvia Sutton sardonically notes, "might have come from Central Casting":

> A father asked to have his son received as an inmate. . . . He informed them that he believed his son to be one of those spoken of in the Bible as "possessed with a devil"; and, when asked what remedial measures he had adopted, replied that he was in the habit of whipping him. The young man was entirely cured, and became subsequently a peddler, in which vocation he displayed so much Yankee shrewdness that he acquired a property of Ten or Twelve thousand dollars.

By the end of 1821, 146 patients had entered the asylum. One hundred and eighteen had left, and there had been six "elopements," as escapes were called. Nine patients died. Twenty-nine were "removed by request" of the administration. Twenty-three patients were discharged as "improved," nineteen "much improved," and thirty-two "cured." The asylum was thriving, already filled to capacity—Bulfinch had designed the wings for one hundred patients—and contemplating expansion. There was just one small problem: The hospital was $20,000 in debt.

Enter John McLean, "a truly noble specimen of Boston merchant," according to a contemporary. McLean was born wealthy, increased his family's fortune, and then, after a series of reverses, found himself in bankruptcy court. But if it is better to be born lucky than to be born rich, it is best to be born lucky *and* rich. A ship of McLean's, long presumed lost, sailed into Boston harbor one day, bulging with precious cargo. McLean promptly invited his former creditors, who had been stiffed in the bankruptcy proceedings, out to dinner at a local hotel and slipped checks with full repayment, plus interest, under their dinner plates. For reasons lost in the fog of time, in 1823, the fortunate, childless trader left a $120,000 legacy to the Charlestown Asylum. The trustees ordered up the traditional thank-you note of the time—a Gilbert Stuart portrait, which still hangs in the administration building*—and renamed the institution after their timely, unexpected benefactor.

Within just a few years of its opening, McLean would change character forever. In 1828, a democratically minded young Massachusetts legislator named Horace Mann delivered a passionate plea to his colleagues for a taxpayer-supported asylum, arguing that "the insane are the wards of the state." Five years later, Massachusetts opened the Worcester State Asylum, which siphoned off poverty cases from McLean. By 1836, according to the newly appointed superintendent, Luther Bell, McLean had become home to "an improved class of sufferers." "This increasing absence of patients from the pauper and humbler ranks of society," Bell wrote, "has rendered the classification, especially of convalescents, far less embarrassing and difficult." "Towns sent their paupers to Worcester," explains historian Sutton, "while wealthier families showed more eagerness to refer mentally ill relatives to McLean, where they would no longer have to fraternize with the destitute."

In 1839, the newly constructed Boston Lunatic Hospital, praised even by the censorious visitor Charles Dickens in his *American Notes,* also began receiving patients, and McLean was well on its way to becoming an upper-class institution. By the middle of the nineteenth century, Sutton writes, "Pauper patients became the

---

*Actually, an excellent copy of the McLean portrait greets visitors when they enter the administration building. A patient attacked and damaged the original in the 1960s; restored, it now hangs in the office of Dr. Bruce Cohen, McLean's president and psychiatrist-in-chief.

exception at McLean. Those admitted, usually in some emergency, were soon transferred to a less costly facility." Turning the cold shoulder to society's less fortunate was the subject of this rationalization in a midcentury annual report:

> Paupers . . . or those in the lower walks of life, whose means are limited, are provided for by various City, County and State Institutions. It has seemed necessary to maintain here, a class of accommodations and a style of living more than simply comfortable, and even in a degree, *luxurious* [emphasis added], meeting the wants, artificial though they may be, of those in a higher social position, and possessed of a competency, who in a state of disease cannot be placed in the best condition for cure, or even present relief, unless surrounded by the comforts to which they have been accustomed.

∽

The glorious setting provided the perfect venue for the increasingly popular moral treatment. Dr. Willard's dunking/drowning regimen—not so far removed from the various coma-inducing therapies that would become popular during the 1930s—was on its way out. Even the theories of Philadelphia's Dr. Benjamin Rush, "the father of American psychiatry," were being questioned. Rush's magnum opus, *Medical Inquiries and Observations upon the Diseases of the Mind,* held that madness was an arterial disease, "a great morbid excitement or inflammation of the brains." An "unrestrained appetite," he wrote, "caused the blood vessels to be overcharged with blood." Thus, he advocated low diet, purges and emetics for vomiting, and hot and cold showers to slow down the overheated metabolism.

And bleeding. Rush was a world-class bleeder, once boasting that he drained 470 ounces from one patient during forty-seven bleedings. Rush was also a tool-bench tinkerer who contributed two mechanical inventions to psychiatry. One was the "gyrator," a rotating board to which patients suffering from "torpid madness" were strapped. Spinning at terrific speeds with the patient's head away from the center, the gyrator pushed blood *into* the brain to stimulate activity. Rush also sold a "coercion chair," called "the Tranquilizer," which supposedly lowered a patient's pulse and blood pressure by holding him or her immobile in the sitting position. A man of many parts, Dr. Rush was also a signer of the Declaration of Independence.

The McLean clientele did receive primitive drug therapy for perceived medical maladies. Purgatives like Epsom salts, calomel, and cochineal were added to food served to overanxious patients. Doctors administered occasional doses of tincture of opium for pain. The colorful eighteenth-century English physician Thomas Dover, perhaps best known for rescuing Alexander Selkirk, the model for Daniel Defoe's Robinson Crusoe, formulated an opium-ipecac compound called Dover's powder that continued to be used well into the nineteenth century. Venesection, purging, and vomiting induced with antimony salts were still used to combat specified ailments. One superintendent dosed five women patients, four of them manic and one paranoid, with tincture of hashish, "an apparently pure and perfect extract" forwarded by a physician in Calcutta. The experiment failed.

Physical restraints were rarely used. McLean's first superintendent, Rufus Wyman, once boasted that "chains or strait jackets have never been used or provided in this asylum." In fact, McLean did use some mechanical restraints, such as hand muffs and leg manacles, and the hospital even bought a knockoff of Rush's Tranquilizer chair. And shortly after buying the Barrell mansion, the trustees opted to build five "strong rooms" to house "raging female patients." In 1836, these were removed after the construction of a "cottage for female patients in seclusion."

But the emphasis was on moral therapy, which Wyman distinguished from medical treatment in an 1830 address to the Massachusetts Medical Society:

The treatment of insanity chiefly depends upon the connection between the mind and the body. If there be inflammation of the brain, or its membranes, it is to be treated as inflammation of those parts. If there be other organic disease, whether of structure or of function, in any part of the body, medical treatment will be required.

But in mental disorders, without symptoms of organic disease, a judicious moral management is more successful. It should afford agreeable occupation. It should engage the mind and exercise the body; as swinging, riding, walking, sewing, embroidery, bowling, gardening, mechanic arts; to which may be added reading, writing, conversation, &c, the whole to be performed with order and regularity. Even the taking of food, retiring to bed, rising in the morning &c, at stated times, and conforming to stated rules in almost everything, is a most salutary discipline. It requires, however, constant attention and vigilance, with the greatest kindness in the attendants upon a lunatic. Moral treatment is indispensable, even in cases arising from organic diseases.

For the well-to-do burghers of Boston, McLean's luxurious rest cure was a lot like living at home. It was in the heyday of moral therapy, under Wyman's successor Luther Bell, that McLean expanded and gentrified its premises. Carpeting, wallpaper, mirrors, open fireplaces, and elegant furniture now graced the halls. In two new houses, built with Appleton money, each patient had a sitting room, a bedroom, and a bath. There were also lodgings for private servants. Here is how Wyman's son Morrill remembered life at his father's institution:

Some of the boarders were quite at liberty to come and go as they pleased. These found their own occupation and amusement; one was a frequent visitor at the reading-room of the Boston Athenaeum, and might have been seen daily among the literary gentlemen who associated there. A constant effort was made to increase the means of occupation and amusement for all. Walking in the airing courts or in the country with attendants, going to church on Sunday, visiting places of interest on other days were the most common. . . . A rowboat upon the Charles River, then attractive and unpolluted, was in frequent use, affording an amusement particularly relished by those who had been sailors. . . .

In summer, excursions in the harbor in large boats gave a pleasant sail, a run upon the islands, a chowder on board, and all the enjoyment of a day away from home. There was bowling, gardening, the exercise of the mechanic arts, books, papers, and various games. Chess was a favorite with some; the physician was an excellent player, and not unfrequently met with a worthy antagonist among his boarders.

Sometimes proper etiquette was therapy enough. A nineteenth-century McLean memoirist named George Ellis recalled the dramatic arrival at Charlestown of a well-turned-out woman in her carriage, screaming that she was engulfed by flames. Superintendent Bell arrived to greet her with the words, "Madam, come with me, and you shall have water." At that, Ellis writes, "She smiled pleasantly, took the proffered arm, and passed into the Asylum as if bent on a stroll through its beautiful gardens."

"By the end of Bell's administration in the late 1850s," writes the historian Sutton, "McLean had evolved into an institution tilted in the direction of the privileged classes, and so it would remain."

∽

Small wonder that when William Folsom, the effete, Phillips Exeter and Harvard-trained apothecary, assumed his duties at McLean in 1825, he found the "crazy people much more pleasant than I expected."

Folsom lived at the asylum's mansion house with superintendent Rufus Wyman and often dined with Wyman's family, as did many of their patients, according to Wyman's son Morrill: "The more quiet also passed their evenings in the physician's family, and always appeared and were treated as gentlemen." Some patients tutored Wyman's children, and one even gave Folsom dancing lessons!

Although he had completed his course work at the Harvard Medical School, Folsom was still a student. In modern parlance, he was interning under Dr. Wyman and attended his mentor's operations both inside and outside the asylum. Folsom's diary recorded three postmortems carried out on McLean patients, only one of which he logged into the asylum case book. Although medically invaluable, postmortem dissections were illegal in Massachusetts before 1830.

Folsom worked hard, rising early each morning to study either the Bible or a medical textbook. He assiduously updated patient records, itself an important therapeutic innovation. And he spent several hours each day socializing with the patients, often at tea time or after dinner. Just twenty-two years old, Folsom kept a diary of the year he spent working in the McLean pharmacy in 1825. It provides a rare window into daily life inside the hospital within just a few years of its opening.

Sunday 8 May
Walk to Norton's road intending to go to meeting at Camb., but ascertained the bells were done tolling, & returned home. Sat in my chamber musing. P.M. [...] Read a little in Bible. Walk with Col. G[oodwin, the steward], met Alex. Hamilton.[...] In wing, reasoned with Amelia M. about being discontented & unruly–rcd advice pleasantly–hope it will do her some good. Miss E. is very jocose–says she recd an invitation to walk this eve. from a *Gentleman of high standing*. Wishes to start in stage for N. Haven tomorrow & will breakfast at *Washburn's Hotel*.
    Bed 10

Sat. 14 May
Rose 5. Walk to Camb. [a walk of about ten miles round trip]. . . . 7:30 breakfast at home. In wings til 11:45 when began to work on Records.

. . . 1, dine—Newspapers—1:45 Records til tea 6:30. Col. G. sat in room after tea—talk of F., B., P., &c [patients]. In wings K. silly & obscene to-day—Mrs. G. excited—With Dr. [Wyman] in S. wing—Ruth S. talked—Girls in III Story pleasant & *orderly*. Dr. amused them with Rabbits of Shadows.

Mo. 11 July
4:30—Kept awake by Dogs & heat from 3:30. Called Col. G. who goes this morn. to Bridgewater. Very hot at 4 P.M. + 92 degrees in Steward's room. Dr. [Wyman] conversed on Intellectual Philosophy last night & this morn. Read a little on Cutaneous diseases in Good [John Mason Good's *The Study of Medicine*]. 10 A.M. visited female wing with Dr. Af-terward til 3 P.M. copying cases. Waiting on company some time. Very hot, can't read. In garden for fruit 6–6:30. After tea walk with P.—shower bath—patients—Journals 2 days—bed

Thurs. 3 Nov.
CHARLES G. of Quincy eloped at tea time from his room, taking out a window and tieing sheets &c together—brick found in room.

Wednesday 9 Nov.
Rose 6. Read Psalms. Visited patients. Walk with attend. & patients to Camb—I called a moment at C's and left directions for Ar. Root saw [sister-in-law] Sarah & S. Eliz. Home 11. records & Patients till eve. Mrs. P died at tea time & I closed her eyes. Mrs. Wyman, with [daugh-ter] Eliz. in my room, talked of Mrs. P. &c

The published version of Folsom's diary even includes the asy-lum's regular weekly menu. Breakfast rarely varied: bread, butter, cheese, and coffee or cocoa. "Supper every day" was Souchong tea, bread and butter, and perhaps toast. Then came

Dinner
Sunday, Soup, meat and vegetables, and bread; or beans or peas, baked, and pudding

Monday, Roasted beef or veal, or lamb, pork or mutton. Vegetables, bread and pudding

Tuesday, Salt beef boiled, vegetables, bread, pudding, or fresh fish, vegetables and pudding.

Wednesday, as on Sunday. . . .

Patients' relatives dropped in often, as did the trustees' Visiting Committee, who took their duties seriously; either Folsom or Wyman escorted them through the premises once a week. In town for the Bunker Hill festivities, the Marquis de Lafayette was supposed to visit the asylum, but he lingered too long at the Massachusetts General Hospital across the river and never showed up. One dignitary who made a point of including McLean on his itinerary was His Highness Bernhard, Duke of Saxe Weimar-Eisenach, who appears in Folsom's diary:

Tues. 2 Aug.

Rose 5:45!!! Attend to B. very sick. the Asylum is this day visited by Duke *Bernhard* of Saxe Weymer, who arrived in a Dutch sloop of war at Boston, a day or two since—also by Mr. Quincy, Mayor, to whom I am introduced by Dr. Wyman.

Aside from presenting an engaging portrait of life at McLean under the old regime, Folsom's diary also contains numerous allusions to his own health problems and his vain attempts to cure them:

Th. 26 May

5:30 Walk—medicines &c. Sick, Dull, sleepy. Read, some, in Wilson on Morbid sympathies, lying on bed. Took *emetic* T. Ant. gr. ii Ipecac gr. vi [two grains of tartarated antimony mixed with six grains of ipecac, to induce vomiting]. . . . Drank cup of tea but vomited it up. Eve. Bright and cheerful, Read Everett's Oration at Concord.

Bed 10

Sunday 11 Dec.
Rose 7. At home all day unwell. Rx last nt. Pil coch. gr. vi last eve., &
Ol. Ric. 6 drams A.M. Operated thoroughly.

Subject to headaches, fatigue, and malaise, Folsom doses himself liberally with the purgative cochineal throughout 1825. "Ol.
Ric." is oil of ricin, derived from the seeds of the castor-oil plant.
One reader of the diary has even suggested that Folsom was a
hypochondriac. Perhaps. But if so, he was a very sick hypochondriac, because he died of unknown causes two years after leaving
McLean, just after his twenty-fourth birthday.

Modern times eventually closed in on the flowering Barrell estate.
What had been a pleasant, rural setting in 1825 had, just fifty years
later, become an urban slum. Four railway lines now girded the
property, and the constant chugging, clanging, and whistling
drove the McLean staff, well, mad. There was always the fear that
an escaped patient might throw him- or herself onto the rails; at
least one did. Filthy metalworking factories, a bleaching and dying
plant, and even a hog slaughterhouse moved into the neighborhood. A local newspaper remarked that "while the [asylum] has
been building up and beautifying within, the opposite has been
going on without. What with slaughter houses, miasmatic
swamps, the area may be said to be slightly unpleasant if not very
unhealthy."

By the time an "eloped" patient died trying to board a freight
train to freedom in 1888, the trustees had already decided to move.

Enter Frederick Law Olmsted, already in the prime of his career,
with three magnificent asylum jobs under his belt: Retreat Park in
Hartford, the Buffalo State Asylum, and the Bloomingdale Asylum outside of New York. Olmsted believed in the curative pow-

ers of sculptured landscape, whether for harried urban dwellers roaming Central Park or for the "harmless monomaniacs" destined to inhabit his retreats or asylums. His designs ran counter to the prevailing notions of asylum construction, which followed the dictates of the so-called Kirkbride plan. According to Dr. Thomas Kirkbride's theory, asylums should be built like hospitals, with large wards attached to a primary administration building. The Kirkbride layout made sense for the public institutions of the time, which had large patient populations and tiny medical staffs. Garrisoned in the central building, doctors could find their way to patients quickly. Its primary disadvantage was that it lumped the curable in with the chronic, the quiet with the excited, and the rich with the poor.

Olmsted and his partner, Calvert Vaux, were designing in a new tradition, which placed wards in separate buildings linked, in the case of Buffalo, by covered porticoes or, at McLean, by underground tunnels. The Olmsted-Vaux arrangement had many advantages for patients. Typically, they enjoyed more space in the mansion-style houses that dotted an Olmsted asylum and were not crammed into one overcrowded men's or women's ward. Furthermore, by the end of the century, asylum administrators realized that patients fared better and even recovered when surrounded by patients with similar maladies. To this end, the decentralized Olmsted-Vaux designs segregated patients by degree of affliction. The "worried well" lived in wards that were more like homes, and they could roam the grounds with appropriate permission. Cynically, but perhaps realistically, the Olmsted-Vaux plans relegated deeply disturbed patients to the periphery of the grounds, where their rantings resounded offstage. Perhaps most importantly, in an era when McLean's "inmates" were finally being called "patients," the Olmsted-Vaux design represented a radical break with the "lunatic hospital" look. After Olmsted landscaped the Hartford Retreat in 1863, director John Butler erected a small horticultural museum on the property and threw open the asylum gates to the public, boasting that the drive which gives the public an opportunity of observing these pleasant changes without exposing ourselves to interruption or intrusion, is exerting a happy influence abroad, in making it evident that the externals of a lunatic asylum need not be repulsive, and may lead to the reflection that its inner life is not without its cheerful, home-like aspects.

Butler summarized the new landscaping program: "Kill out the Lunatic Hospital and develop the home!"

The Olmsted-Vaux design, as implemented by McLean's deep-pocketed trustees, created some very comfortable living quarters. The Belmont plan called for 160 private patient rooms, a slight decrease from the Somerville census. Twenty of those rooms were private apartments, with parlors, bedchambers, and bathrooms. The first two houses built, Appleton and Upham, sported large, oak-paneled reception rooms with views over the surrounding countryside, intimate dining rooms with large windows, and deep, open fireplaces. The kitchens, the laundries, the heating, and the plumbing and sanitary facilities were the most modern available. The weekly cost of a McLean stay quadrupled, from $5 to $20. Among other comforts, that fee financed a 2:1 patient-to-staff ratio; publicly supported asylums had a 10:1 ratio or worse.

Indeed, as historian Silvia Sutton notes, for patients who hailed from a certain stratum of Boston society, McLean looked a lot like home:

> If, in the fall of 1895, an innocent wayfarer had trespassed on McLean's territory in Belmont, he might have believed himself to have strayed into some curious residential development for very affluent people with excessively large families. He would have been astonished to discover that what he was looking at was, in fact, a hospital for the care and treatment of the mentally ill. . . . The initial impression, to quote one observer, was of "gentlemen's country residences irregularly dispersed in a pastoral landscape."

How did the patients fare in the move? The brusque change of environment could have been severely destabilizing, but the McLean administration had planned ahead. The Somerville patient count had been drawn down to about 120, partly by freezing admissions and also by discharging chronic cases deemed too unsteady for the change. Closer to the actual date, many of the remaining patients began to worry that they would be paraded through the streets of Somerville and Cambridge, subject to taunts and jeers from onlookers. But the transition was handled with aplomb. During the month of October 1895, small groups of patients were invited to go for carriage rides, a common group recreation. But these carriage rides ended up inside the elegant new grounds in Belmont. "Then, one day," writes medical historian Grace Whiting Myers, "much to their surprise, they found that they were all in the new McLean; and as for the public, they read about it in the newspapers after it was all over."

3

The Mayflower Screwballs

The insane asylum seems to be the goal of every good and conscious Bostonian, babies and insanity the two leading topics. So and so has a baby. She becomes insane and goes to Somerville, baby grows up and promptly retires to Somerville.

Clover Adams, writing to her father in 1879

In modern times, McLean would become famous not only as a therapeutic locus but also as a literary and artistic landscape. Even in increasingly grubby Charlestown, which was starting to attract unsavory factories and slaughterhouses, McLean had its share of what we might now call celebrity patients. Two of Ralph Waldo Emerson's brothers lodged in Charlestown. Robert Bulkeley Emerson was retarded from birth and spent many years in and out of the hospital, as the family's finances permitted. When not at McLean, he boarded in a rooming house and sometimes helped out on Israel Putnam's farm in Chelmsford. More tragically, in

1828, another brother, Edward Bliss Emerson, suffered an unexpected nervous breakdown and was sent to McLean. Edward's institutionalization weighed heavily on his older brother Ralph, who was somewhat in awe of Edward's accomplishments. The boy had finished second in his Harvard class, unlike Ralph Waldo, who finished thirtieth out of thirty-nine; Edward had just been accepted into law practice with Daniel Webster. It is from Ralph Waldo Emerson's pen that we have one of the first descriptions of the shock a family member experiences when visiting a loved one in the mental hospital:

> He has been now for one week thoroughly deranged & a great deal of the time violent so as to make it necessary to have two men in the room all the time. . . . His frenzy took all forms; sometimes he was very gay & bantered every body. . . . Afterward would come on a peevish or angry state & he would throw down every thing in the room & throw his clothes &c out of the window; then perhaps on being restrained wd. follow a paroxysm of perfect frenzy & he wd roll & twist on the floor with his eyes shut for half an hour.
>
> There he lay—Edward, the admired, learned, eloquent, thriving boy—a maniac.

Edward died of tuberculosis at age twenty-nine. Robert lived in the Boston area until he died at age fifty-two.

Emerson had another McLean connection, one that he documented more thoroughly than his familial ones. At the recommendation of Miss Elizabeth Peabody of Salem, Emerson befriended a young Harvard Greek tutor and poet named Jones Very. Even by the standards of Emerson's eccentric inner circle, Very was odd. At the beginning of the 1838 academic year, Very shared with his students and his supervising professor the news that he was the Son of God and that the Second Coming of Christ was at hand. This was news Harvard apparently was not ready to hear. The tutor was shipped back to Salem, where he played a similar trick on his friend, Miss Peabody. Invading her parlor early one Sunday morning, he placed his hands on her head and announced that he had come to baptize her with the Holy Ghost and with fire (Matthew III, Chapter II).

"I feel no change," Miss Peabody told Very.

"But you will," said Very. Soon afterwards, one of his cousins had him forcibly removed to McLean.

Very spent only a month in the hospital, lecturing the patients on poetry and Shakespeare and regaining some inner calm. Upon his return, the Salem locals credited McLean's superintendent Luther Bell with saving the tutor and poet "from the delusion of being a prophet extraordinaire." They thought this had been accomplished by righting Very's "digestive system," which had been "entirely out of order."

Emerson embraced Very upon his release, inviting him out to his Concord home and even editing a book of his poems, gratis, for publication. But some members of Emerson's coterie still bristled at the presence of this high-maintenance divine. Bronson Alcott, an oddball himself, praised Very as "a mystic of the most ideal class . . . a phenomenon quite remarkable in this age of sensualism and idolatry" but complained that Very was "insane with God" and "diswitted in the contemplation of the holiness of Divinity."

Then, almost as dramatically as he had acted up, Very inexplicably calmed down. "Very no longer felt God-directed," according to Emerson's biographer John McAleer. "The result was he had become a dull fellow." He returned to Salem, where he lived quietly for another thirty-two years. "His kindly, careworn face," McAleer writes, was "a melancholy reminder to those who saw it of the afflatus that had, for a brief moment, exalted him before it departed forever."

Emerson immortalized his "treasure of a companion" in his famous essay "Friendship," published in 1841:

> We parry and fend the approach of our fellow-man by compliments, by gossip, by amusement, by affairs. . . . I knew a man who under a certain religious frenzy cast off this drapery, and spoke to the con-

science of every person he encountered, and that with great insight and beauty. At first, all men agreed he was mad. But persisting, he attained to the advantage of bringing every man of his acquaintance into true relations with him. . . .

To stand in true relations with men in a false age is worth a fit of insanity, is it not?

∽

Patient records at McLean are now more closely guarded than they were thirty years ago, when the record room was open to all staff doctors and some valuable Sigmund Freud letters went missing. The diaries of therapeutic regimens, sometimes spanning decades and comprising hundreds of pages, make for fascinating reading. Some records, like that of Boston's John Warren, are works of literature, as insightful and revealing of mid-nineteenth-century Boston as James Boswell's diary is of Samuel Johnson's London.

This John Warren was the son of the above-mentioned John Collins Warren and grand-nephew of the hero of Bunker Hill. Not only did John Collins Warren lead the unsuccessful subscription for the new hospital in 1810; he is also credited with first using ether as a medical anesthetic. A famous painting by Robert Hinckley depicts Dr. Warren operating with ether under the Bulfinch-designed dome at the Massachusetts General Hospital. To the surrounding doctors and gawkers, Warren memorably proclaimed: "Gentlemen! This is no humbug!"*

---

*Warren was the first doctor to use ether successfully, but he did not discover it. A quarrel over credit for the discovery of ether's anesthetic properties supposedly sent one of the claimants, Dr. Charles Jackson, to McLean. The story goes as follows: Jackson believed that his former lodger, an entrepreneur named William Morton, had stolen the anesthesia idea from him. Legend has it that when Jackson happened across Morton's gravestone in Mount Auburn Cemetery and saw him credited as the "inventor and revealer" of anesthesia, he suffered a mental breakdown and was sent to McLean. "Jackson's face no longer looked human, and the cries he uttered were unlike human cries," one writer recounted. "The creature that cried and thrashed with its limbs in Mount Auburn Cemetery was unchained madness." Actor Julius Tannen

John Collins Warren had several sons, the eldest being the future McLean patient John. But the father favored the next-born, Mason, who followed in his footsteps and became a surgeon. Mason, however, proved to be sickly, and, not so surprisingly, his father's regimen of purgings and archaic medicines did not do much to improve his health. The father often assigned his eldest son to care for the beloved younger brother, and during a therapeutic trip to Cuba, John Warren's raucous and undisciplined behavior landed him in trouble with tavern keepers, prostitutes, and the local police. On his return in 1841, his father packed him off to McLean, where he was to spend the next thirty-four years of his life. John's name was expunged from the family Bible; he had become an official nonperson. One modern psychiatrist who has reviewed Warren's record notes dryly that if he was not crazy when he was admitted, he was certainly crazy by the time McLean was through with him.

Here is the log book entry for John Warren's first night at McLean, April 19, 1841:

Admitted age 33; unmarried.

No business, nor property in his own right.

This gentleman is the eldest son of Dr. John C. Warren of Boston.

(continued from page 38)

depicted Jackson dancing maniacally on Morton's grave in the 1944 movie account of the ether controversy, *The Great Moment.*

Because anesthesia was one of the world's most important medical discoveries, the ether wars rage on. Two medical historians, Dr. Richard Patterson and Richard Wolfe, now argue that Jackson *was* unfairly denied credit for pioneering the use of ether as anesthesia and that it was Morton's supporters who spread false accounts of Jackson's dipsomania and lunacy. In the twentieth century, Jackson's family jawboned McLean's Franklin Wood into furnishing them with a summary of their forebear's medical record. (Jackson had conducted some ether experiments at McLean to see if the gas calmed severely disturbed patients. Those experiments failed, but after his breakdown, the grateful trustees allowed him to live as a "guest" at the asylum for seven years until his death in 1880.) Even though Jackson's death certificate cited the cause of death as "insanity," Wood reported that Jackson had suffered a stroke, followed by aphasia, causing loss of speech and memory. "There is nothing in this record that would indicate in any way that Dr. Jackson was intemperate in the use of alcohol or that he was a 'raving maniac,'" Wood wrote.

His history in one sense is soon told & he has been a true son of *Ishmael*, with "his hand against every man and every man's hand against him." Such has been his strange and erratic course of life, that it may safely be doubted whether he *ever did a sane action*. The only satisfactory explanation of life is he was *constitutionally insane* and *never recovered*.

To enumerate his peculiarities of thinking, feeling and acting would be to describe his whole life and therefore impossible. Naturally brilliant and active, he was never disposed to apply his mind. Impatient, restless, mischievous, yet no settled malice, disobedient to his parents, yet of kind and tender feelings. Fond of broils, fights, and daring deeds yet not intemperate and noisy.

He seemed determined to have his own way and succeeds by stern, daredevil manner with "actions suited" to his words. Was always in trouble, skulking about to avoid detection: chased by sheriffs for assaults, and debts: unhappy at home and shunned and detested abroad. Once *stabbed* a man and *fled* his *country*. While in Europe spent all the money his friends could furnish and all he could *borrow* and get on the Credit of his father. Of late has been boarding in the *American House* [now called the Parker House], living high, drinking Wine, Beer & Smoking Cigars, running up Bills at Tailors, Barbers, Livery stables, etc.

Yesterday was the first time that he ever discovered to his friends any *palpable* delusions. He then thought a *young lady* was *desperately* in *love* with him and *had sailed for Europe without disclosing it to him*. He also imagined he heard *screeches* and *cries* in the house where he was boarding and that he had *injured some one*, perhaps *his mother*. He also has the idea he was *pursued* by *enemies* [and] that he had been *poisoned*. Was *suspicious, wild & fearful*.

Warren's first few months in confinement proved to be quite eventful, punctuated by manic episodes, paranoid outbursts, and even an escape attempt:

April 20
Slept but little during the night, and attempted to *injure* himself by

springing headforemost from his bed onto the floor. Sprained his muscles about the neck and was prevented from further injury by his attendant.

April 21
In painful distress because he thinks he must have committed some *outrage* in the city. Full of delusions. Thinks he is accused of *murder* and *theft*, & other crimes.

June 15
Mother died. Was fearful he "should go distracted" did not know but "his conduct had killed her." Could not weep. Went home to see her on condition of not [reprimanding] his father—could not keep his promise. Writes insane letters.

Aug. 2
Went to walk with a new attendant, decoyed him into the city. Went into a shop and made his escape. Took his razor with him but did not use it improperly.

Aug. 5
Was returned today by a constable—found him at *Nahant*, had driven about from place to place *chiefly in the night*.

Oct. 1
During the past month, has been more civil & quiet but his delusions are at times strong—hears false sounds, as of screams of females suffering and crying for help—thinks the superintendent said to him on blowing his nose, "those are dear blows"—thinks the viscid secretions of his mouth are purulent matter and is exceedingly alarmed.

Oct. 15
Treated the supervisor rudely—was put in his room and promised never to repeat it. Was surprised to find that anyone dared to lay hands upon him.

Oct. 20

Made an attack upon a fellow boarder because he started at him as he thought—threatened to strike with a chair was overcome by the other but not injured—is now removed to the W. Gallery. Lays it much to heart—can see no necessity for "such solitary confinement."

Nov. 8

Today attended the Probate Court to defend himself from being put under Guardianship—exposed his delusions to the court—got angry—and in coming out to the street attempted to make his escape—was caught and returned but is yet civil.

Dec. 1

Much as formerly—attempted to make a key from the brass of his umbrella—Never very social—pretty civil—*aristocratic.*

Of course.

Warren's file shows months on end with no entries or just a brief notation, "in status quo." His demeanor remained unpredictable: He was at times the gentleman, "musing and playing his flute," and at times he was impulsively violent, "[kicking] about the furniture & breaking the chairs." He heard voices, he entertained delusions, and he acted strangely, wrapping his socks over his shoes in order, as he explained, "to prevent the strength from going out of his legs." In 1843 and 1844, he believed whores were persecuting him and threw his chamber pot at them. He was denied the use of a knife and fork. When the trustees showed up for a visit, he complained that he was being abused by the attendant, who "excited his private parts by some magnetic influence." He then demanded "his release on the ground he is perfectly sane."

For the next several years, Warren fell into a routine. He was reclusive; every other afternoon, he walked into Charlestown with an attendant following a few feet behind him. He spent about $10 a month on "books, paper, clothing and eatables." He also bought his own crockery because he believed the institutional plates and cups were unclean. Warren could be an irascible customer, and some shopkeepers barred him from their premises. What is striking is the lack of recordable or noteworthy incidents and the frequent observation that Warren was faring quite well. Years went by without mention of a destructive incident:

Nov. 26, 1847
Has gone through the summer without any sickness.

April 2, 1848
Taking the past year together it has been a more comfortable one than he has ever passed since under the charge of the asylum.

Jan. 1852
There has been no change for several years.

Dec. 29, 1853
No change. Good health.

Oct. 2, 1860
The past year has been without incident or change.

May 30, 1861
As unsocial and determined to be exclusive as ever. Health uniformly good.

Nov. 20, 1863
Has had uninterrupted health since last date and there has been no change in his mental characteristics, or habits.

Nowhere in his record do we find the suggestion that he return to his family's care. His family's interest in him seems to have been negligible. In 1863, one of his brothers paid a call, "not having seen him for five or six years before." The man thoughtfully left John some Tract and Temperance Societies publications. One day in 1866, the warder noted that "he expressed a wish that 'Dr. J. Mason Warren would come and take him out of here.'" There is no record of any further communication on this matter. Now almost twenty years into his stay, John was avoiding the trustees and timed his visits to Charlestown so he could be absent during their weekly sweeps through the asylum. Warren was slovenly and paid little attention to his appearance. He took wine daily and had a healthy appetite, but as time progressed, he ventured out of his room less and less. "Few of our household pursue a more uniform & unvaried life than he does and in none is there less change noticed," we read. For years, the entries read as follows: "General health uniformly good. . . . General health good. . . . Idem."

Two events of consequence occurred in the years before his death. First, he allowed his attendant to walk next to him rather than "several rods behind" during his occasional visits to Charlestown. And second, he started to manifest symptoms of a *folie de grandeur*. He said more than once that he owned Appleton, the ward where he was staying, and that "they would not be able to run it if he was not about to manage affairs." In fairness, Warren had spent far more time at McLean than any of the three superintendents he knew.

In August 1875, in his sixty-seventh year, Warren fell sick with a painful cough. To alleviate his symptoms, he swallowed "medicinal" brandy with mustard powder on the side. He also imbibed essence of peppermint, spiked with morphine, to relieve pain. Over the course of several months, his health began to fail. On December 4, 1875, John Warren's lengthy incarceration came to an end: "Sank quite rapidly during the night and died this morning a mere skeleton with nothing to keep it together but an indomitable will."

The cause of death was an abscess of the right lung. John Warren had lived through the Civil War, the opening of the western frontier, and the era of the railroad on a tiny plot of land atop a hill in Charlestown, Massachusetts.

In two-inch square advertisements placed in The New Yorker *and in* the Harvard and Yale alumni magazines, McLean still boasts of its "unsurpassed discretion and services." Of course, McLean guaranteed discretion for its patients; in some cases, it may have guaranteed complete secrecy. Some doctors believe that patients have been able to expunge any record of their stay from the McLean archives, which were often subject to prying eyes. One example often cited is that of Edward William "Ned" Hooper, the longtime treasurer of Harvard University and brother of Clover Adams, Henry Adams's wife. Both of Ned's siblings, Clover and another sister, Marian, committed suicide, and at age sixty-two, Ned decided to join them. He flung himself out of the third-floor window at his Beacon Hill home, barely falling short of a spiked iron fence that would have decisively ended his life. The *Boston Evening Transcript,* not necessarily the most reliable diagnostic source, concluded that Hooper suffered from "a temporary mental derangement." Whatever the case, he ended up at McLean and died there two months later of pneumonia, according to Clover Adams's biographer Otto Friedrich. Yet a doctor who went hunting for Hooper's name in the McLean archives failed to find it; nor did he find another or even a pseudonymous patient admitted at the same time in similar circumstances.

Which leads us to one of the most-researched footnotes in American intellectual history: Did William James, the brilliant, depressive, "father of American psychology" ever sojourn at McLean? Several doctors and even a former director of the hospital have assured me not only that James stayed at the hospital more than once but also that they saw his name on the patient record list. In his 1975 book *Freud and His Followers,* historian Paul Roazen states categorically that "James was perhaps the first of the Cambridge, Massachusetts intelligentsia to make personal use of the services of McLean Hospital." "I had it straight from [the psychologist] Erik Erikson," Roazen told me. "There was no hesitation. He would have known because he was very interested in James." But other equally knowledgeable sources, while not denying that James may have been a patient, swear there is no record of his having been there. Some doctors insist that he may have been admitted under an assumed name, but, as in the case of Ned Hooper, there does not appear to be a pseudonymous male patient who answers to William James's description. Historian Linda Simon, author of a recent James biography, was allowed to peruse the McLean intake logs, with names deleted, for the winters of 1870 and 1871, when James suffered what he called the "great dorsal collapses"—physical agony from back pain, coupled with immobilizing depressions—and fell off the map. There were yawning gaps in his correspondence then, and many friends and family members assumed he had left on a long trip. But if he was at McLean, Simon found no trace of him. "I found nothing that correlated with the facts of James's life during that period," she reported. "She's got the dates wrong," Roazen states bluntly. "James would have been there towards the end of this life."

I recall the distinct sense of elation and discovery when the late Dr. Ruth Barnhouse told me in 1997 that as a young resident at McLean, she had stumbled upon William James's case file. "In those days all the charts were easily available," she said. "I used to read the records when I was on duty overnight, and I found his." But Barnhouse told Simon essentially the same story, corroborated by James's godson William Sheldon,* who also worked at McLean. Sheldon was not the only James family member to place the great philosopher and psychologist inside McLean. William James's son Henry has testified that a famous anecdote in his father's landmark *Varieties of Religious Experience* about a terrified Frenchman suffering a shocking catharsis inside an asylum ("After this the universe was changed for me altogether") actually hap-

---

*Sheldon lives in the collective memory of medical history as the theoretician of "constitutional medicine," which argued that physique and posture provided clues to temperament and intelligence. It was thanks to Sheldon that incoming freshmen at Harvard and Yale were photographed nude from the 1940s through the early 1960s, by way of testing his since-discredited hypotheses.

pened to James himself. The family patriarch, Henry James Sr., once referred to his son's "experience at the Somerville Asylum," but this is ambiguous because in his professorial capacity, William escorted medical students into McLean on teaching visits. Simon further speculates that William James's own son William, who also suffered from depression, may have been a patient at the hospital, thus contributing to the general confusion.

The quest for proof of James's hospitalization continues. Michael "Mickey" James is William James's only surviving grandson and lives in a modest ground-floor apartment in Boston's Back Bay neighborhood. A sculptor of tirelessly cheerful disposition—his answering machine greets callers with a boisterous "how-de-do!"—Mickey has assumed the role of point person in the James versus McLean affair. He agreed to inquire about his grandfather's records after receiving a letter from Ignas Skrupskelis, the University of South Carolina philosophy professor who is collecting and editing the correspondence of William James. "I have over the years heard rumors that there are William James letters at the McLean Asylum, Belmont," Skrupskelis wrote Mickey in 1992, requesting his assistance. "The Asylum claims that all patient records are confidential and will not even state whether or not there are any letters."

Mickey forwarded the Skrupskelis letter to the then-director of McLean, Dr. Steven Mirin. "As it's been a hundred years and more since the W.J. records were closed, neither ethically nor legally can I imagine why his letters, if any, should be denied a reader's scrutiny and pleasure," James wrote. "William would have agreed, don't you think?" Mirin may well have had other things on his mind. The hospital was going through an especially dark period, with deep deficits and staff layoffs prompting talk of closing it down. Whatever the case, James soon received a response from archivist and registrar Terry Bragg explaining the hospital's long-standing policy of complete patient confidentiality, in perpetuity. Only in cases where all the surviving relatives agree to the release of a case file will the hospital allow a copy to leave the premises. Mickey, who has no children, dutifully collected ten letters from his own nieces and nephews. Then a friend pointed out that to satisfy McLean's request for "an explicit statement from each surviving heir," he would also have to amass the signatures of all the descendants of his two uncles, William and Henry, and of his aunt Peggy. For now, the project is hanging fire, although shaking loose the McLean documents—if any exist—is hardly Mickey's top priority. "It's all very interesting to think about," he says. "But there's not one shred of actual evidence that William James was ever there."

4

The Country Clubbers

It was a country club in the best sense of the word.
What's wrong with having a country club?
Dr. Robert Coles

Soon after McLean opened its doors in Belmont, the now-defunct American Journal of Insanity dispatched Dr. Henry Hurd of Baltimore, himself a mental hospital superintendent, to peruse the new facility and report his findings. Hurd hailed the new hospital as meeting all the "requirements for successful treatment of patients of a comparatively well-to-do class." Designed for patients "accustomed to luxuries and comforts at home, to whom seclusion, pleasant, tasteful, and refining surroundings . . . were essentials to cure," the new McLean "marked a distinct advance in the treatment of curable insanity in America." Hurd continued enthusiastically:

In the new McLean Hospital the buildings have been so arranged as to prevent the occupants of one from coming in contact with those of

another. . . . Beyond this the interior arrangements of individual buildings furnish complete seclusion to excited patients, so that it is possible for them to go through an attack of insanity without seeing any
other patient. The buildings resemble gentlemen's country residences
in a natural park rather than the structures of a large institution.

The trustees had hired the city's most eminent institutional architects, Fehmer and Page, to design the several wards and the stable, and H.H. Richardson's disciples Shepley, Rutan, and
Coolidge to create the administration building. "Always buy the
best" was the watchword of Boston's blue-blooded dowagers, and
their husbands followed suit. The burnished-copper rain gutters
still hang from the marble cornices of North and South Belknap
Halls. Roofs were copper or slate, never shingle. Every patient's
room had a fireplace, ample closet space, bath, and toilet. The second hall built for men, Upham Memorial Hall, was larger than
many hotels but accommodated only nine patients, each in a luxury suite with a sitting room. In every ward, the rooms were
soundproofed with layers of plaster inserted in between upper and
lower flooring. There would be no patients loitering aimlessly in
corridors. "These corridors are not used as parlors," Hurd wrote,
"but serve only as passages to parlors of good size, which are
sunny corner rooms in almost all cases. It is everywhere sought to
obtain a domestic style of construction and homelike effects."

What was life like at McLean at the beginning of the century?
The neatest portrait of the new Belmont hospital emerges from
the pen of Earl Bond, a twenty-nine-year-old medical school graduate who took a job as "junior assistant physician" at the newly
landscaped facility in the summer of 1908. Bond went on to enjoy
a distinguished career in psychiatry, both as an officer of the
American Psychiatric Association and as an administrator and
doctor at the Institute of the Pennsylvania Hospital in Philadelphia. His son Douglas and grandson Thomas both became psychiatrists; Thomas was an attending physician in Belmont for
eighteen years. After his retirement at the age of eighty-three, Earl

Bond started work on a memoir of his psychiatric career, beginning with his halcyon years at McLean. When Bond wrote about the hospital, he have might been describing a secluded village or a baronial ski resort:

> The road to the hospital climbed a steep hill until it reached the lower side of a long, open plateau and then followed the edge of the grassy field to the administration building. . . . The porches and windows of this building gave unobstructed views of several miles of the countryside to the west. Trees shut out views to the East and South and the little town of Waverley lay hidden behind a shoulder of the hill.

Fifty years after leaving the campus, Bond still remembered the large, indoor gymnasium, the two tennis courts, and the "rough and ready golf course" with its final, ninth green terraced right in front of the administration building. (The seldom-inspected cup at the little-used ninth hole was a favorite dope stash for the 1960s generation.) But even this description understates the recreational facilities. The new hospital had *two* indoor gymnasiums, one for men and one for women, each with its own billiard room and bowling alley.

The new McLean had beds for 100 male and 120 female patients. They were attended by three doctors, including the superintendent George Tuttle, and by three assistants like Bond. For most of the century, the campus would be split along north-south and male-female lines, the "Men's Division" occupying the northern tier and the "Women's Division" the south. The nurses were mainly women; because of a local labor shortage, many of them were recruited from high schools in Maine and Nova Scotia. The first female physician would not appear on the grounds until shortly before World War II. Because of a resignation, Bond quickly became chief of the Men's Division, and he visited each male patient every day. Twice a week he joined the grand tour of the hospital with Tuttle and the other doctors, who looked in on all the patients.

The ever-cheerful Bond clearly enjoyed his five-year-long stay at McLean. He and his new bride moved into a newly purchased, white clapboard farmhouse near the Mill Street gate, and he whiled away his leisure hours playing first base on the softball team alongside the burly male ward attendants. The staff was congenial. Although Tuttle held himself somewhat aloof in his formal residence, the doctors and various service chiefs enjoyed their meals together at two large tables in the ground-floor dining room of the administration building, where many of them lived. But professionally, Bond realized that he had settled into a medical backwater. He was interested in psychiatry, partly because his sister-in-law had overcome a mental illness and partly because he had enjoyed a two-month-long elective tour of McLean while in medical school. But not one of his Harvard Medical School classmates went into the field, and even within psychiatry, jobs at mental hospitals were not highly prized. When positions opened up at McLean at the turn of the century, few qualified applicants expressed interest in them. One research job was filled by a "highly recommended chemist who had come from Germany" and who liked to entertain fellow staffers while piloting his sailboat around Boston Harbor. He turned out to have sailed extensively in the Halifax and Portland, Maine, harbors as well. "Shortly before World War I broke out, he 'happened' to go back to Germany," Bond reported, "and we wondered rather late in the day if he had been a spy."

The patients hailed primarily from the upper strata of Boston society; they were men and women whom poet Robert Lowell would later brand "the thoroughbred mental cases." Bond treated a man who fantasized that he sailed his yacht along the streets of Boston; another young patient had landed in Belmont after forging checks at his Ivy League college. "This was doubly unwise," Bond wrote, "because his father was president of a bank." "A man with one of the most honored names in Boston was admitted to my service," Bond recalled, "because his family found that he had lost his memory":

He had been made guardian for many widows and orphans. It turned out that he had lost all the properties entrusted to him. A reconstruction of events brought out what must have happened. He would open a deposit box, take out the stocks and bonds, stuff them into his pockets and go to his office. There he would find his pockets uncomfortably full and empty them into the waste basket and the maid would put them in the trash can.

One can envision the coupon-clipping Brahmins frog-marching this hapless custodian up the hill to McLean, and double-quick!

By just one year, Bond missed treating one of the most extraordinary patients ever to enter the hospital: Stanley McCormick, the son of Cyrus McCormick, inventor of the combine harvester and one of the richest men in turn-of-the-century America. Stanley was both typical and atypical of the kind of patient checking into McLean in 1906: atypical in that he was far wealthier than even the carriage-trade clientele then finding its way to Belmont. He was so wealthy that his family would eventually hire away his McLean doctor and caretakers and relocate them to a private estate in Santa Barbara, California. But in other ways, Stanley was all too typical, because in the end he could not be helped.

Cyrus McCormick had three sons and two daughters. Of the three boys, Stanley was the youngest, the "sensitive" one. His mother, Nettie, a devotee of patent medicines and religious revivals, shuttled him among private schools in Chicago and generally smothered him with maternal care—and with strictures; when her children misbehaved, Nettie locked them in a dark closet. When Stanley was still a teenager, his sister Mary Virginia suffered a psychotic breakdown and never appeared in society again. He attended Princeton, played tennis marvelously, and studied art.

Stanley talked about becoming an artist and even attended an art school in Paris after his college graduation. But family pressure directed him to the McCormick Harvest Machine Company (later International Harvester), where he sat on the board of directors and occupied various executive posts. Stanley was bright and quick with numbers. But he struggled in his assignments. He agonized over decisions; underlings, sometimes frustrated by weeks' delay in the most routine deliberations, circumvented him and complained about his behavior to his brothers. Judging from the numerous psychiatric reports written during Stanley's forty-one years of mental illness, he suffered partly from what we now call an obsessive-compulsive disorder. His McLean write-up notes that "he kept six or eight different weights of underwear and he had a certain range of temperature for each set, and every morning it was almost impossible for him to decide what the temperature was going to be and which set of underclothing would be the proper one."

Tall, handsome, and athletic, the young Stanley McCormick never felt particularly well. Working for the fast-growing family harvester business overwhelmed him. More than once, a family doctor diagnosed "nervous prostration," and Stanley even bought a 45,000-acre ranch in New Mexico to serve as a sanctuary from the press of worldly concerns. One day in the summer of 1903, he reported looking at his face in a mirror and seeing only a blank. The next day, motoring through the ocean-side town of Beverly Farms on Massachusetts's swank North Shore, he happened upon his childhood acquaintance, Katharine Dexter.

Katharine, who, like Stanley, was twenty-eight years old, was not the same little girl he had known in dancing school sixteen years before. The daughter of a prominent Chicago lawyer, she was attractive, self-possessed, and about to enter her senior year at the Massachusetts Institute of Technology. Because of the many hurdles placed before the handful of women at MIT, Katharine took eight years to get her degree. Stanley wooed her assiduously, if unconventionally. He was in one of his socialist phases and wanted to discuss the plight of the working class during their dates. Katharine, one of the wealthiest and most socially conscious women of her generation, was bored to tears. Worse still, he discussed his own failings in intimate detail. During one of their secret engagements, he confessed that he was a compulsive masturbator and had even made a leather harness that he wore at night to keep his hands away from his genitals. Although Katharine appreciated Stanley's intelligence and love of the arts, the confessional, self-deprecating Stanley was more than she could stand. She wanted a real courtship—flowers, trips to the theater, fun! In the words of Stanley's patient history, Katharine was "a girl who preferred light to shadows." After her senior year, she fled to her family's chateau in Switzerland—once occupied by Voltaire and by Napoleon's brother Joseph Bonaparte—to be rid of Stanley. Incredibly, Stanley accosted her on the wharf in New York and told her that a leading urologist had given his genitalia a clean bill of health. Katharine sailed alone.

Stanley pursued her to Europe, and the rest is psychiatric history. He was handsome, temporarily clear-minded, and in love with her; Katharine capitulated. Against the better judgment of both families—Nettie, informed by telegram, flopped on her bed and wept for days—Katharine and Stanley married in Geneva in September 1904. Although the honeymoon lasted for nine months, the marriage was never consummated. (The presence of their respective mothers during parts of the trip could not have helped.) Most nights, Stanley refused to come to bed, scribbling letters until dawn. When he tried to make love with Katharine, he failed, blaming either his youthful masturbation or a sexual encounter he may or may not have had with a Parisian prostitute several years earlier.

After the marriage, the couple lived apart, with Stanley working for Harvester in Chicago and Katharine living in Boston. In 1906, Stanley's dysfunctions came to the fore. He was forced to resign from the family company and rejoined his wife at her home in Brookline, a comfortable Boston suburb. On account of his nerves, Stanley and Katharine spent that summer at a cottage in Maine. Once back at home, in the words of his doctors, "the patient's wife reminded him that he had had a good rest, and that he was improved. Accordingly, she told him that there was no reason he should not discharge his physical obligations; an heir was wanted." That effort, in late September, came to naught. Stanley went downhill rapidly and initially consulted the Dexters' friend, the eminent Harvard neurologist James Jackson Putnam, who advised that he take fencing lessons and study German to distract his mind. A few days later, Stanley assaulted a dentist, whom he had allowed to pull a tooth without using anesthesia. Then he attacked an elevator operator, and he subsequently dragged a German tutor out of his office and into the McCormick home to administer the prescribed lessons. On the night of October 16, Katharine took him to McLean.

With the admitting doctors, Stanley was alternately pugnacious and delusional: "While looking into vacancy, he exclaimed, 'Jack London! I'm glad to see you.' When no one had spoken he repeatedly said, 'Who is calling me?' When restrained in bed he shouted 'To Windsor! To Windsor!'" Katharine explained to the doctors that Stanley's appeal to Jack London was not random: "She thinks at this time he was thinking of turning over his fortune to the socialists," a notion that probably shocked Stanley's family a good deal more than it shocked her.* On the admission form, the doctors noted under "Heredity," "All the family of nervous temperament, mother eccentric, sister insane." The diagnosis on admission was "Manic-depressive? Dementia praecox? Fixed ideas?" Two years later, when two male nurses wrestled Stanley into a private railway car bound for his new home in Santa Bar-

---

*Stanley had attempted to unionize the ranch workers on his New Mexico spread, to no avail. The McLean doctors record that "the patient had been so far interested in Socialism as to have given some money, surreptitiously, to the 'Cause.'"

bara, the diagnostic question marks remained. "Diagnosis on discharge: Psychopathic-inferiority + manic-depressive insanity? Dementia praecox?"

The hope in the fall of 1906 was that a period of complete rest and "detension" in one of the luxurious suites in Upham Memorial Hall would restore Stanley's spirits. And for a period it did. In late October, he experienced "a period of steady improvement," according to a summary of the doctors' notes. "Patient perfectly clear, natural in attitude, showed good insight, and discussed his symptoms frankly. . . . Gaining in weight and sleeping well." He received birthday gifts in early November and wrote daily letters to Katharine, who visited him often.

But in what would soon become a pattern, his clear periods were interrupted by episodes of abnormal behavior. His wife's visits sometimes upset him; in conversations with his doctor, Gilbert van Tassel Hamilton, Stanley confessed that he had been impotent in his marriage. He remarked that his nurses were calling him a dog, and in response, he put his plate on the ground and lapped up his food with his tongue. He masturbated openly and flew into a rage when the nurses tried to stop him. Then a major setback occurred in December. Even though he admitted that he could feed himself, he chose to be fed through a tube forced down his esophagus. He attacked a doctor and tried to hang himself with the drawstring of his pajamas. That was viewed as a feeble suicide gesture because he was never left alone.

By the winter of 1906, Katharine and the McCormicks had already squared off in what would prove to be a forty-year battle for control of Stanley's care and of his estate. Faced with evidence of Stanley's decline, both sides agreed to appeal to Swiss-born Adolf Meyer, then viewed as the preeminent psychiatrist in America. Meyer journeyed from Manhattan to Belmont, examined Stanley, and delivered the bad news: Nettie's youngest son was becoming catatonic.

Meyer, who would later become even more prominent as chief of Johns Hopkins' prestigious Phipps Clinic, seemed to have the

Stanley McCormick case pretty well nailed. He reported that the patient

> had an early center of trouble in the excessive development of frustrated sex-functions. He had an excessive sensitiveness in his adjustment to his mother, the business responsibilities and rather abstract standards of a socialist and moral-religious system of accounting for everything. Under the strain of special conflicts the patient went through courtship and marriage, only to find himself utterly unable to cope with the new problems, not at all sexually and socially only with a hopeless expense of energy.

The December setback and Meyer's bleak diagnosis engaged Stanley's family in the worst possible way. It was Katharine who had had him committed and who for a time visited him every day. A trained biologist, she demanded and received daily, written reports from superintendent Tuttle, and she monitored Stanley's care closely. But Nettie and her daughter Anita Blaine were quite wary of Katharine's education and firmness of mind. "She thinks like a lawyer," Anita remarked. "Her mind has the characteristics of a man's mind," Nettie told a friend, and neither comment was intended as a compliment. Nettie, of course, blamed the assertive and self-confident Katharine for her son's breakdown. "[We] feel that heretofore in his times of perplexity and uncertain health K did not evince devotion to him, and did not, in illness, tenderly watch over him—and has not appeared that she was proud of him," she wrote to a friend. Meyer, stupidly, enmeshed himself in the family drama. As a paid consultant to the McCormicks, he began agitating for Katharine to divorce Stanley, an outcome fervently desired by Nettie and her other children. Even the McCormicks' lawyer knew that Katharine had a strong claim on Stanley's fortune, which did not prevent him from offering her a generous financial settlement to divorce her husband and leave him to his family's care. Katharine spurned the buyout offer.

Inevitably, Katharine and Nettie clashed over Stanley's care. Katharine opted to stick with McLean's genteel regimen, or moral treatment, for two years. McLean's superintendent Tuttle opined that Stanley "will pull out of it if he can be kept quiet and given time." Nettie was much more critical of the McLean doctors' approach. During the first few weeks of her son's convalescence, she sent her family doctor, Henry Favill of Chicago, to Waverley to check up on Tuttle and Hamilton. Nettie wanted to bring "the great Vienna doctor [Richard von Krafft-]Ebing," or France's Valentin Magnan* into the case. Favill let her down gently, saying in a letter that no foreign doctor could work miracles in absence of a precise diagnosis: "I think that the matter would have to be determined by individuals in this country." When Stanley experienced his brutal relapse in December, Nettie claimed that "the doctors who are relied on to know things were incautious—and unaware of the brittle condition of Stanley's mind." The following month, Nettie wrote to Dr. Tuttle from the Watkins Sanitarium in Glen Springs, New York:

I find benefit to my nerves from electricity applied to me through the warm water of the bath given here. The battery is at the head of the bathtub. The bath is a warm tub bath—not hot. The electricity produced a simple, pricking sensation. Can you give such a bath to Stanley, I mean have you the bathtub equipped with such a battery?

I also have benefited from static electricity—I sit in a chair and a wire arrangement shaped just like a simple crown, or cap, is swung above my head after I sit down and the current is turned on, until a pricking sensation is produced. It is the most sleep producing treatment I have here. It *soothes*.

Have you appliances to give this static electricity?

---

*Krafft-Ebing was famous for his textbook *Psychopathia Sexualis;* both he and the equally prominent Magnan believed that insanity was brought on by hereditary degeneration, a detail probably unknown to Nettie.

At the end of the letter, she wrote, *"I am not hearing as I wish from my son."* In fact, the doctors had cut her out of the reporting loop. Tuttle and Stanley's attending physician, Hamilton, were sending their medical notes only to Katharine and the "reasonable" family member, Anita. This did nothing to silence Nettie, who wrote to Hamilton, "Can you not devise a purely *oxygen cure* for him—that is—live in a cloth room—with one side removed—adjacent to a *closed* room, with fire warmth—then *live* in the cloth room, having it warmed if needed, but live in a *cloth room* most of the time. He gets but little oxygen—the real article." Or, "How would it do to begin with rubbing *just one leg,* at first with cool water—not too cold—*just one leg below the knee,* then, next day, the *whole leg.* . . . The method of doing only one member at a time does away with the argument that application of cool water would throw him into excitement."

When Stanley was clear, which was much of the time, he was the typical McLean patient, puttering around the golf course, pedaling the Zander machine (an early version of the stationary bicycle), or regaling his attendants with stories of his hunting trips in Maine. On May 13, 1907, the anniversary of his father's death, he addressed a letter to his mother:

> I have thought of you today as we have indeed been together on this day many times in love and thought. . . . I have played 24 holes of golf today. Started out before breakfast with one of the nurses named French & we had six. This morning Dr. Hamilton and Mssrs. MacKillop & Tompkins who is also a nurse here had a round of the course in a foursome match. This afternoon the two latter and I played another round. I have been doing some work in charcoal in between my outings.

But Stanley's moments of clarity alternated with long periods of catatonic inactivity and with outbreaks of violence. In the spring of 1907, he hid in the bathroom of a neighboring suite rather than meet with his wife. A few months later, he assaulted Katharine, prompting Dr. Hamilton to curtail all visits from women. Katharine and Anita agreed on a radical intervention: They decided to relocate Stanley to a family-owned estate, Riven Rock, in Montecito, California. The gorgeous stone mansion overlooking the sea had initially been purchased as a home for Mary Virginia, who had since been moved to a private sanitarium in Alabama. Katharine lured Hamilton, who was doing research on primate sexuality, to the West by endowing the nation's first freestanding primate research institute on the estate grounds. Similarly, she convinced two of McLean's male nurses to pull up stakes and spend what proved to be the rest of their lives caring for her husband.

Stanley spent the next thirty-nine years at Riven Rock.* Hamilton drifted away, to be replaced by McLean's chief research pathologist, August Hoch. The ensuing psychiatric quadrille will become a familiar tale in later chapters of this book. Just after Stanley left McLean, the family paid a small fortune—$2,000 a week in 1908 currency—to bring Emil Kraepelin, the world's most famous psychiatrist, to Stanley's bedside. Kraepelin's lengthy report essentially recapitulated Meyer's conclusions of the previous year, with one exception. Whether out of politeness or conviction, Kraepelin held out a slim hope for recovery, noting that Stanley was suffering from an "active disease," catatonic schizophrenia, as opposed to a "terminal condition." As for treatment, Kraepelin had no suggestions to improve upon the Hamilton-Tuttle regime imposed on Stanley from the first day of his breakdown: "rest treatment ... should be continued ... continuous baths ... warm packs" and so on. Kraepelin was aware that some voices might be calling for Stanley to be psychoanalyzed. Stanley himself said twice that "he would like to have Dr. Freud visit

---

Riven Rock is the name of a 1998 novel by T. Coraghessan Boyle that dramatizes Stanley's and Katharine's plight during his lengthy California exile.

him." But Kraepelin ruled that out: "Any definite mental treatment is not practicable at the present time, since the patient is essentially inaccessible." Freud never came, nor did Carl Gustav Jung, whom Nettie approached by letter in 1912.

The tragedy of Stanley McCormick seemed interminable. Forbidden by the doctors from meeting with her son, the dying Nettie McCormick traveled to Montecito in 1923 to gaze at him through a crack in his bedroom door. In 1929, in a lawsuit publicized in every major American newspaper, Katharine sued Anita and her brothers for sole guardianship of Stanley, claiming that Stanley's new attending physician, Dr. Edward J. Kempf, was bilking the family for $150,000 a year and doing her husband no good. Katharine had soured on the potential success of talk therapy and had begun her search for a possible biochemical explanation for Stanley's disease. The previous year she had endowed the Neuroendocrine Research Foundation, tasked with exploring the role of hormone imbalances in schizophrenic patients. The lawsuit provoked a media circus. "Freudism as Used on Harvester Heir Is Fought by Wife," the *New York World* reported of the trial taking place in Santa Barbara. "She Contends Sex Psychology Treatment Alienates Love of Stanley McCormick; Seeks to Oust Dr. Kempf of N.Y. from $150,000 job." The coverage continued:

> Psychoanalysis—the sexual psychology of Sigmund Freud—is the central issue in the fight in the International Harvester McCormick family for control of the incompetent multi-millionaire Stanley McCormick, who now lives the life of both prisoner and potentate on his vast seaside place at Riven Rock. . . .
>
> Mrs. Katharine Dexter McCormick, his wife, who is fighting to wrest control of her husband from his brothers and sister, is aiming mainly to discharge Dr. Edward J. Kempf, noted New York psychoanalyst, who came to Santa Barbara in 1927 to devote his entire attention to the "mad McCormick," at a salary of $150,000 a year.
>
> Picturing psychoanalysis as a fantastic and exploded theory, her counsel, former Secretary of War Newton D. Baker . . .

And so on. Katharine eventually paid $500,000 in legal fees, with little to show for it. She did get Kempf fired, but the court forced her to continue sharing Stanley's guardianship with the McCormick family.

Katharine never remarried. Dividing her time between Montecito, where she monitored Stanley's care from a neighboring estate, and Boston, she used the considerable Dexter-McCormick fortunes to become one of the nation's leading philanthropists, endowing the pioneering birth-control research of Margaret Sanger and Dr. John Rock, who conducted some of the first field tests of the birth-control pill. When Stanley died in 1947, his lawyers produced a will scribbled out in longhand in 1906. It proved to be one of the "letters" that Stanley was writing at night during his honeymoon instead of attending to his wife. He left her everything, an estate then valued at about $35 million. After four decades of open warfare with her in-laws, Katharine finally won Stanley back. At the elite Graceland Cemetery in Chicago, she had Stanley's body laid to rest in the Dexter plot, far removed from the McCormicks.

Katharine died in 1967, leaving huge bequests to the Stanford University Medical School, the Chicago Art Institute, the Chicago and Boston symphonies, and Boston's Museum of Fine Arts. All of the gifts, including the priceless impressionist paintings she and Stanley had collected on their honeymoon, were made in the name of her late husband. The largest beneficiary in her will was her alma mater, the Massachusetts Institute of Technology. Toward the end of her life, she wanted desperately to build a dormitory for women; there was none on the MIT campus. In fact, she had been paying taxi fares for female students to commute to her beloved "Tech" from housing across the Charles River. By 1960, she managed to get the plans for Stanley R. McCormick Hall under way. "I am particularly happy to be able to provide a dormitory on the Tech campus for women students there," she wrote to her friend Sanger. "This has been my ambition for many years but it had to await the oral contraceptive for birth control." She lived to see the first wing dedicated in 1963. The second wing was completed just after her death. She was buried in Chicago, next to the handsome man she had met during a chance encounter at an ocean resort sixty-four years previously.

∽

The amenities at the new Belmont location were extraordinary. In addition to the "architected" riding stable, McLean comprised a working farm, with separate beef and dairy barns; two piggeries; extensive vegetable and flower gardens; a working apiary for honey; and apple and pear orchards, which are still visible on the left when one drives into the hospital. (The orchards are slated for removal to make way for luxury housing.) Fish and meat came from Boston's Quincy Market. Otherwise, patients mainly consumed what came from McLean itself: fresh water from a prodigious spring and donuts and rolls from a bakery that turned out one hundred loaves of bread a day. The food was by all accounts very good. "We catered to patients," a former steward recalled in the hospital's official history. "If the patient did not like the lamb we served for dinner and asked for lobster, we gave lobster. They could afford it. Appleton House [the men's ward] was the Ritz Carlton."

As time progressed, it became less and less economical for the hospital to bottle its own milk or slaughter 2,000 pounds of pork a week during the spring and fall. The nation's need for manpower put an end to the dairy business during World War II. In the 1944 annual report, Franklin Wood noted that "it was necessary to dispose of the herd of cows this year because we were unable to find or keep dairy hands." The herd had roamed the campus for fifty years, and he lamented their departure: "It was a sad affair."

For those disposed to enjoy them, there were cultural opportunities in the form of "regular weekly entertainments." In the mid-

1930s, Wood selected a few for special mention: "Mr. Frank, with his 'Seeing-Eye' dog Buddy, visited the hospital, showed his pictures, gave an interesting talk, and allowed us to see Buddy in action." Another visitor, Stephen Corey, a member of Richard Byrd's second polar expedition, "gave a most instructive talk and showed us a duffel bag full of equipment, explaining the use of the various articles." Patients could even study art. A group of high-minded ladies converted a portion of the women's gymnasium into an art room, stocking it with fifty original oil paintings (including a Guido Reni of questionable provenance), watercolors, and reproductions of the great religious works of Venice and Florence, mostly for teaching purposes. The small gallery also housed copies of the Venus de Milo, the Hermes of Praxiteles, and about a dozen other marvels of antiquity. Patients could peruse the annotated catalog and attend art-appreciation classes if they so chose. The donors expressed their hope that when the restorative powers of Olmsted's delightful landscape might wane, art would fill the breach: "In the beauty of outward surroundings on this hill-top, the ministry of Nature is manifest, even if, in suffering, one can not always realize it. Often—certainly in times of heat or cold or storm, when Nature's power of helpfulness is suspended—it is hoped that within, after some simple fashion, Art may minister charm and serenity."

But the most powerful signal to the city's well-to-do that McLean was offering a level of service not customarily found in mental institutions was the construction of the first of several free-standing "cottages for one patient," completed in the summer of 1896. It was a cottage in name only, not unlike the sprawling, flagstone "Berkshire cottages" that graced the landscape of Edith Wharton's New England novels. The five-bedroom, two-story colonial revival home faced west, overlooking a terraced garden and the rolling hills of Belmont. On the ground floor, one found an entry hall, a dining room, a living room, a spacious sun room, a kitchen, a pantry, and a china closet. Each of the two ground-floor bedrooms had a separate bath and a three-foot-by-five-foot closet. Upstairs, there were three smaller bedrooms, with smaller closets, all sharing one bath—the servants' quarters. Also on the second floor were two storerooms and a linen closet. All this was for one patient and the requisite support staff.

The cottages proved to be popular with McLean's aristocratic clientele, who could enjoy the comforts of home as well as full-time access to some of the best medical and psychiatric care in the country. Although each arrangement was slightly different, a wealthy Boston family—the Schraffts and the Shaws were two well-known examples—would typically pay for the construction of the cottage and deed it to McLean in return for lifelong care of a disturbed relative. An elderly man I know recalled visiting his cousin Nellie in one of the cottages, where her furnishings and maids had all moved in. As a young boy, "I had to go have tea with her once, and she introduced me to all the portraits on the walls." One cottage was built to replicate a woman's Brookline home. Legend has it that she was transported in her sleep from Brookline to McLean, woke up in the hospital, and lived the rest of her life in the comfortable and appealing surroundings. Architects Peabody and Stearns designed the Arlington Cottage with four-foot-thick fire walls to assuage the pyrophobic fears of the patient whose family paid to build it.

∞

During the period between the two world wars, McLean ran by the book, in this case two small, spiral binders compiled by chief psychiatrist Kenneth Tillotson and director Franklin Wood. The binders sat on Wood's desk and governed every aspect of hospital life. Wood was a fussy man, a professional administrator who had done a good job overseeing construction of a new wing for the Massachusetts General Hospital and so had fetched up at McLean. A dapper Rotarian of no scholarly attainment—"He knew

everything that went on, except what went on in patients' heads,"
Dr. Paul Howard told me—Wood was not even a psychiatrist. But
he was an occasionally tyrannical stickler for detail, and all the details necessary for running the hospital were stored in his meticu-
lously typed rule book, awaiting execution. Some excerpts:

DRIVES: A nurse who accompanies a patient on drives must cover
her uniform with a coat and wear a hat.

SMOKING: Smoking in bed is not allowed, except in the case of a
patient who is confined to bed because of physical illness.

MORGUE: If a patient expires between 7:00 P.M. and 7:00 A.M.
give post mortem care and leave body in room with window open and
room door locked until morning. In the morning, one man nurse with
one chauffeur will take body to morgue by hospital truck.

The lengthiest entry concerns the proper care and feeding of
one Miss "Julia Bowen," the not-terribly-crazy offspring of a
prominent Boston family. As Tillotson describes it, Miss Bowen's
life as a "madwoman" in one of McLean's sumptuous cottages is
one we might all envy:

Miss Bowen does not live according to the strict rules and regulations
of the wards but leads a fairly natural and free life and has special permissions. As nurses and supervisors are used to the strict ward rules
and would not know in what way Miss Bowen was supposed to live
and the special permissions which she has, the following statements
and permissions have been listed and signed by the doctor.

Miss Bowen goes in and out of the house to the piazza and garden
and dooryard frequently.

Miss Bowen looks after her garden, garden supplies and imple-
ments herself with such help as she requests.

Miss Bowen goes to bed and gets up freely as she feels the need,
within reason, and reads when she feels like it—night or day.

Miss Bowen has baths once or twice a day as needed and shampoos
her hair to suit herself.

Miss Bowen can have her razor when she needs it, as well as her scissors, nail file, hair tonic, etc.

Miss Bowen has permission to have and use electric stoves, heaters, flat-iron, curling iron, curling iron heater, percolators, waffle iron, electric fans, humidifiers, blower, diffuser, and sewing machine.

Miss Bowen takes care of her birds . . . or superintends their care. She diffuses them to delouse them.

Miss Bowen studies music, vocal and instrumental (piano), practices and goes to lessons. She sometimes has her teacher come to the house.

Miss Bowen goes to the theater, movies, concerts and other entertainments.

Miss Bowen goes on boat trips.

Miss Bowen goes to the shore and goes in bathing.

Miss Bowen has permission to go out Sundays as well as week days.

Miss Bowen has permission to take a taxi and go for a ride.

Miss Bowen has permission to mail letters herself to the people whom she is allowed to see or do business with.

Miss Bowen has permission to go to the dentist, oculist, and skin specialist.

Miss Bowen has permission to have a veterinarian if her birds are taken ill.

Miss Bowen has permission to have ice cream and things from S.S. Pierce, Breck, and the tailor delivered to the cottage.

Miss Bowen may have friends to meals.

Miss Bowen may have certain friends visit her without special permission or yellow slips, either before or after 7:00 P.M. (note list of such friends).

It is not a "transfer" for Miss Bowen to sleep in some other room in her cottage. She may do so if it is inconvenient for her to sleep in her bedroom on account of papering and painting or repairs.

Approved and signed by:

Kenneth J. Tillotson, M.D.

Class considerations permeated every aspect of life at the hospital. In 1940, two McLean staffers, Dr. Abraham Myerson and Rosalie Boyle, presented a paper to the Massachusetts Psychiatric Society entitled "The Incidence of Manic-Depressive Psychosis in Certain Socially Prominent Families." The authors announced, "We have studied up to now 20 families which might legitimately be called socially important"—all of them at McLean. "The reasons for this selection are obvious, when one considers that . . . the psychotic members of distinguished families of New England have found this the most convenient institution for the care and treatment of their condition." The authors stop short of naming names like Adams, Lowell, and James, but just barely: "There have been several governors of Massachusetts . . . a great many Federal judges, including chief justices of the Supreme Court . . . philosophers of international importance," and so on and so forth.

The fifteen-page paper is unintentionally comic, analyzing the phenomena of intermarriage and intramarriage among Boston's First Families: "People of great importance and ability tend to become socially intimate by a sort of social chemotaxis [a fancy word for a chemical combination]." The writers explain that the rich and powerful, wary of fortune hunters, engage in "proper mating," which in turn causes "caste levels to be developed, even in a democracy." The authors note that each time a family member shows up at McLean, he or she purports to be the first person of the line to have mental problems. "The first thing we discovered was that the statement 'family history negative' has fundamentally no meaning," the researchers report, adding, "We present here 8 charts in which the statement 'Negative family history' appears concerning a patient at McLean Hospital, and in which the true facts as obtained merely by a survey of the hospital records themselves indicated a definite, in some cases marked, incidence of mental disease in the family group." When it comes to mental illness, even the best people lie.

The patient write-ups from this period might be taken verbatim from the novels of John Marquand, the mid-twentieth-century chronicler of Boston's declining aristocracy. (Marquand complained about the high cost of McLean when his own son had to go there.) The lengthy case file for "Priscilla Jenkins," who married into the outer branches of a well-known literary family, focuses as much on her breeding, social connections, and mildly dysfunctional family life on Hilliard Street in the chic section of Cambridge as it does on any illness she might have had:

> The patient is the product of a socially prominent Boston family that has had financial security of such nature that all the children were able to secure anything they desired. . . . The patient was educated in France for one year, then back to boarding school for about eight years and then spent a year in Italy. She speaks French quite fluently and learned Russian during the War but has since forgotten it. She has studied dancing, mainly ballet, since the age of eight.
>
> The patient has never had to work for her living, but has danced frequently as a professional. She danced at the New York World's fair, Vincent Club shows, a year and a half at the Latin Quarter in Boston, and taught dancing at private schools in Wellesley for a year and a half.

Before the present era of "five-day admissions," when psychiatrists had the time to delve into a patient's background, they routinely summoned as many family members as possible to the hospital to discuss a case. We pick up the thread of Priscilla's story in the words of one of her brothers, "a neatly dressed, well-educated and very cooperative individual":

> In 1939, the patient ran into a fellow, whom the family unanimously decided was a bum as he had a bad record and came from a poor family. The family attempted to make it plain and tactfully as they could to her that she was barking up the wrong tree. They found that each

thing they said was pushing her more toward him. . . . She then married him and it turned out worse than the family had expected as he came back from overseas and spent his money on various women. Mrs. Jenkins then came back to live with her mother.

The first unhappy marriage ended, after two children, with a quick trip to Reno. Then Priscilla bumped into her second husband, like her first a product of Harvard College, a former paratrooper with some shrapnel souvenirs lodged inside him. His brother-in-law called him a "two-fisted fellow . . . a red-blooded fellow, likes to drink." Priscilla liked to drink too, up to six cocktails a day, which may have contributed to her psychological difficulties. A miscarriage of her new husband's child severely depressed her, and the ensuing cycle of treatments aggravated her condition. After seven sessions, she became terrified by electric shock treatments. Then she became addicted to the barbiturates prescribed to calm her down. A doctor prescribed Empirin, a codeine-laced analgesic, and amphetamines to get her off the phenobarbital, but these only contributed to her agitation. During this period, her chart notes that "she did give up her alcoholic consumption and drank nothing but three or four cans of beer a day." It turned out that her druggist had continued selling her sleeping pills, and she had never really been unhooked anyway. Her brother recounted that her husband had not exactly urged her to seek psychiatric help. "The husband would respond that he saw 'Snake Pit' [the gruesome Olivia de Havilland movie that depicts life in a particularly hellish asylum] and according to that, you should leave them alone." Priscilla's second husband, in the clubland vernacular, had proved to be unsound, her brother said:

He drinks quite a bit, however, he is one of those fellows that can take two or three drinks in the morning and two or three drinks in the afternoon and run his business O.K. I am of the opinion that his mind is so fluttery that he can't settle down and get a job. Not normal not to be doing something. He says he wants to write a book.

The same doctor who spoke with her brother interviewed the husband, too:

The husband is a tall, black-wavy-haired, masculine individual who gives one the impression that he is not particularly upset about his wife's condition, and that he is rather indifferent to her problems and tends to shrug them off. He is very anxious to cooperate as to interviews and is quite willing to leave the problem of duration of hospitalization and treatment in our hands.

He conveys the idea that he is active in some business (without telephone) and has sort of dropped much of it to take care of his wife. She denies his working since marriage and says that they mostly live on her income, except for a small part that he has. He would lead one to believe that he is the model husband with over solicitous care and tenderness, but he is very insecure in his relationship with his wife, due to the financial arrangement.

Priscilla Jenkins was discharged after two weeks. Her McLean doctor, Douglas Sharpe, wrote that she "had shown marked physical improvement since her hospitalization. She has gained weight, slept without medication, and has not complained of any somatic problems since her two epileptic convulsions on February 5, 1949, which were probably due to drug withdrawal. . . . All the various complaints she presented on admission have disappeared. She frankly stated that she presented these problems in order to gain attention and sympathy." The prognosis, Sharpe reported, was "guarded."

Priscilla Jenkins died at age fifty of lung cancer.

5

The Search for the Cure

I remember one of my supervisors, the famous Abraham Myerson, when we asked about treating depression, saying: "Look, we give them Dexedrine for depression, and then they get elated. Then you give them phenobarbital to calm them down. They ricochet between mania and depression." And that's really what it was, with electric shock, wet sheet packs, and hot tubs all thrown in.

Dr. Edward Daniels

*Addressing the American Psychiatric Association in 1933, Presi*dent James May bemoaned the state of the profession. Few medical schools employed professors in the field of psychiatry. Mental illness, May said, was "a medical playground" in which neurologists, neurosurgeons, and psychiatrists competed with gynecologists and ophthalmologists in speculations on the causes of psychoses. From about 1930 until the introduction in 1954 of Thorazine, the first usable antipsychotic drug, the curative landscape resembled not a playground so much as the Wild West. Every few years, a new sheriff would ride into town, promoting a new wonder cure that eventually yielded to the next, short-lived fashion.

In the 1930s, for instance, a Trenton psychiatrist named Henry Cotton pulled patients' teeth and removed their large intestines to cure mental illness, which he believed to be caused by "autointoxication." (Stanley McCormick's psychiatrist, the well-regarded Adolf Meyer of Johns Hopkins, hailed Cotton's work as a "remarkable achievement of the pioneer spirit.") For a while, fever was thought to be restorative for mental patients, especially for the stiff-gaited victims of general paresis, the physical and mental paralysis that accompanied the advanced stage of syphilis. Some hospitals—McLean was not one of them—kept malarial mosquitoes or diseased rats on hand to bite treatment subjects and induce fever. Others injected blood from fever victims into the paretics, who crowded the mental hospitals until the discovery of penicillin. For the ostensible purpose of boosting patients' white blood cell count, some doctors injected horse blood into their subjects' lumbar cavities, mixing the blood with spinal fluid. Then sleep therapy, or "prolonged narcosis," came on the scene. In theory, a week-long, drug-induced nap would help restore a patient's exhausted nervous system.

In 1941, two McLean doctors, John Talbott and the bumptious Kenneth Tillotson, reported encouraging results from a therapy they called hypothermia. Like Dr. Willard's drowning regimen of a century and a half before—and like the various shock therapies coming into use during the twentieth century—the hypothermia cure reduced the body to a near-death state by lowering the patient's body temperature. It was not hibernation, the doctors emphasized, and was decidedly not refrigeration. "We object to the word refrigeration," they wrote, "because it implies that the object treated is refrigerated and that the temperature is reduced considerably lower than is compatible with life." Their modus operandi and their conclusions seem comic to us now, all the more so because they cited an 1805 cold-water dunking of an English convulsive as an important precursor for their experiment. But Talbott and Tillotson produced two important results: Four of the ten patients whose body temperatures they lowered by twenty degrees or more for periods of up to sixty-eight hours (!) showed marked improvements. The mental state of one sixteen-year-old boy cleared to the point where he could leave the hospital and go home. And one patient, a forty-six-year-old male paranoid schizophrenic whom they kept cold and semiconscious for fifty hours, died when his lowered blood pressure never came back again. The doctors injected him with adrenaline and caffeine, to no avail. "It is hoped that this would not have occurred," Talbott and Tillotson wrote. But it did.

The procedure sounds, well, chilling. After sedating the schizophrenic patients with a barbiturate (Nembutal) and a muscle relaxant (Evipal), the doctors wrapped them in special blankets manufactured by the Therm-O-Rite Products Company of Buffalo, New York, through which they circulated a refrigerant. A stomach tube pumped glucose into the patient to keep him or her alive, and a thermocoupled rectal thermometer transmitted body-temperature readings every other minute. The patients were garden-variety catatonic, paranoid, and hebephrenic (the "laughing disease") schizophrenics. One young woman, a twenty-five-year-old medical student, had already received *Dauernarkose* (continuous sleep), insulin shock, metrazol, and typhoid vaccine therapies before coming to McLean. She had an unusual reaction to the cold: Her mental acuity cleared when her body temperature was more than ten degrees below normal, and she then reverted to her disturbed condition as the thermometer approached 98.6. She had three hypothermia treatments and was classified as a success, although she remained at the hospital. Overall, the doctors claimed success in four cases, temporary improvements in four others, and no discernible effects in the remaining two. The younger patients with shorter histories of mental illness responded better than the older patients; it was the oldest patient who died.

Talbott and Tillotson derived a "modicum of hope" from their work: "The results would seem to be at least equally as promising as insulin and metrazol in the treatment of schizophrenia," they wrote. They felt compelled to add that "hypothermia does not cause morphologic damage," meaning bodily harm. That is true, unless one includes death by cardiac arrest.

∽

A kinder, gentler form of therapy was the various water treatments that had been administered to mental patients since the end of the eighteenth century. (A young psychiatrist once asked Paul Howard, who joined the McLean staff before World War II, why patients comported themselves better after hydrotherapy treatment. "Don't you always feel more relaxed after a nice, warm bath?" was Howard's commonsensical reply.) The 1922 McLean nurses' manual lists no fewer than seventeen different hydrotherapy regimens, from the foot bath to the shampoo. Most are categorized as "tonic baths" and administered in the "hydriatic suite" in the basement of the women's gymnasium. Here are a few of the treatments and a partial list of the illnesses they were supposed to assuage:

Hot Air Bath	Alcoholism, manic depression, dementia praecox (senility)
Electric Light Bath	Same
Vapor Bath	Same
Salt Glow (an eight- to twelve-minute rubdown with salt crystals)	Huntington's chorea, involution melancholia, multiple sclerosis
Fomentation (application of moist heat using a thirty-inch-square piece of white woolen flannel)	Same, plus cerebral syphilis, paralysis agitans, etc.

Revulsive Sitz Bath ("As patient arises from the bath, a pail of cold water, 80 deg., is splashed upon the hips.")	Neuralgia
Pail Douche ("Have water at three temperatures in pails holding several gallons. Dash the contents of each pail over the patient in quick succession.")	Good tonic treatment
Wet Mitt Friction (loofah or white mohair)	"Invaluable in inaugurating hydrotherapy in the psycho-neuroses"
Neptune Girdle (apparently a variant of the cold wet sheet pack, placed around a woman's waist)	"Employed extensively in the treatment of the psychoneuroses"

One of the most common hydrotherapies was wrapping the patients in cold (forty-eight to fifty-six degrees Fahrenheit), wet sheets. These so-called packs were used to pacify agitated patients up through the 1970s. In 1922, the packs' effect was divided into action ("sensation of chilliness . . . cooling of the skin . . . shivering") and thermic reaction ("chilliness disappears . . . skin become warm . . . muscular relaxation occurs"). Hypothermia was of course a risk: "If there is any unusual paleness of the face, blueness of the lips or shivering, the patient . . . should be warmed by the application of hot water bags to his sides and feet. He should also be give a hot stimulating drink. (A teaspoonful of whiskey in hot water is considered good because whiskey dilates the blood vessels in the skin.)"

Another ubiquitous remedy was the "continuous bath." According to the nurses' manual, the prolonged bath could be "administered for hours, days, weeks or months." "In some hospitals [and this is a tip-off that we are *not* speaking about McLean], it is customary to keep the patients in the tubs 18 hours daily and some very disturbed patients are kept in the baths without removal for periods of 2 or 3 weeks."

Director Franklin Wood's desk notebook of course codified every last concern about the continuous baths, from the proper temperature (ninety-four degrees Fahrenheit) to the possible dangers: "1. Heat prostration; 2. Chilling; 3. Scalding; 4. Drowning; 5. Convulsions." The following instruction would indicate that some patients did spend day-long cycles in the baths: "If a patient is very noisy, restless, or flushed, or if the pulse rate is 88 or more rapid, supply an ice collar. Sponge the face of each patient with cold water once or twice during the bath. Omit during sleep."

∞

The real action, however, was in the shock therapies—insulin coma, metrazol, and electric—which were widely used at McLean and elsewhere at midcentury. "All the theories attempting to explain how these treatments worked proved to be wrong," writes Elliot Valenstein in his delightfully readable psychiatric history, *Great and Desperate Cures,* "and, as they were stated, so vague as to be impossible to take seriously."

Insulin coma was discovered by accident by the colorful Viennese physician Manfred Joshua Sakel, who claimed to be a direct descendant of the twelfth-century rabbi, physician, and philosopher Moses Maimonides. Sakel unintentionally gave a diabetic mental patient an overdose of insulin, lowering her blood sugar to the point where she fell into a coma. When she emerged from unconsciousness, she felt considerably better. In clinical trials, Sakel reported an astonishing 88 percent success rate, and he even treated the famous Russian dancer Vaslav Nijinsky. Success, of course, is always relative in psychiatry; Nijinsky did not figure in the lucky 88 percent and was not able to resume a normal life after Sakel's treatment.

Insulin coma caught on quickly in the United States, as did metrazol shock, which had precisely the opposite effect on patients. After examining the cadavers of epileptics and schizophrenics, a Hungarian researcher named Joseph Ladislas von Meduna had concluded that epilepsy and schizophrenia were mutually antagonistic. Thus, theoretically, an induced epileptic seizure would "cure" a psychotic patient. Meduna found that a synthetic chemical called metrazol would send patients into the desired convulsions. (Other doctors similarly enamored with the epilepsy-schizophrenia connection tried injecting epileptics' blood, drawn immediately after a seizure, into mental patients. These conjectures have little basis in scientific fact.)* Meduna, like Sakel, Freud, and many ambitious European doctors before him, eventually made a U.S. landfall, and popularized his treatment around the country.

Metrazol shock naturally led to electroshock therapy, which also caused patients to go into convulsions. "Medical electricity" was nothing new. Scribonius Largus, who lived in the first century A.D., treated the Roman emperor's headaches with electric eels. In the eighteenth century, a French physician used electroconvulsive therapy on a patient with psychogenic blindness. In his early neurology practice, Freud experimented with low-grade electric shock, "only to find [it] grossly ineffective and lacking any sound foundation," according to one history of psychiatry. "Freud realized [perhaps "hypothesized" would be a better choice of word] that the electric-current therapy was only a form of covert suggestion

---

*In the 1960s, a researcher named Heinrich Landolt also noticed that epilepsy and schizophrenia are reciprocally related, and he floated a theory of "forced normalization," which holds that epileptics' mental afflictions lapse during a seizure and reassert themselves when the seizure is being treated. More generally, many schizophrenic patients do become temporarily "clear" when subjected to extreme stress. The classic examples are a medical emergency or a fire on the disturbed ward; patients usually respond to rescuers' commands. So an induced epileptic seizure, electric shock, or even dunking in frigid water sometimes awakens the responses of "blocked" patients. But the underlying psychiatric disorder almost always reappears in short order.

and had no lasting therapeutic effect." But its widespread use on psychiatric patients originated in Italy in 1938, when the police commissioner of Rome sent an apparently dazed schizophrenic to doctors Ugo Cerletti and Lucio Bini for treatment. Cerletti and Bini had seen hogs killed at a Rome slaughterhouse after being stunned with electric current. They experimented with the hogs to determine a nonlethal dose of current; this prompted them to theorize that the brain produced a "vitalizing substance" called "acro-amines" in response to a convulsion. The police commissioner's referral provided them with their first human subject.

Valenstein describes the ensuing opera buffa:

> When the current was applied to his head, his body jolted and stiffened, but he did not lose consciousness. Clearly, the voltage was too low, and they decided to try again the next day. Overhearing the two doctors, the patient said, "Not another one! It's deadly!" As those were the only comprehensible words they had heard the patient utter, they ignored his protests and decided to try again immediately with a higher current.

We pick up the story in Dr. Cerletti's words:

> We observed the same instantaneous, brief, generalized spasm, and soon after, the onset of the classic epileptic convulsion. We were all breathless during the tonic phase of the attack, and really overwhelmed during the apnea as we watched the cadaverous cyanosis of the patient [who is turning blue]. . . . Finally, with the first stertorous breathing and the first clonic spasm, the blood flowed better not only in the patient's vessels but also in our own. There upon we observed with the most intensely gratifying sensation the gradual awakening of the patient "by steps." He rose to a sitting position and looked at us, calm and smiling, as though to inquire what we wanted of him. We asked: "What happened to you?" He answered: "I don't know. Maybe I was asleep." Thus occurred the first electrically produced convulsion in man, which I at once named electroshock.

Electroshock therapy, too, was quickly accepted in the New World, mainly because it was deemed easier and safer to administer than the insulin or metrazol shocks. Just three years after the Rome experiment, McLean reported that forty-three patients, eleven men and thirty-two women, had received the new treatment. Psychiatrist-in-chief Tillotson noted that nine of the patients showed no apparent benefit. Thirty-four of them "responded with clinical improvements of varying degree and duration." Of these, twelve were able to leave the hospital. As was often the case with all of the shock regimens, the patients hurt themselves. Even when securely strapped to a gurney, their bodies sometimes exploded into dramatic and extreme contortions.* Five patients suffered compression fractures in their spine. Two others dislocated their jaws. Rooting behind a bank of file cabinets in his office, McLean archivist Terry Bragg once showed me the first electric shock apparatus purchased by the hospital, a Reiter Electro Stimulator manufactured in Italy in 1938. It was a chunky, briefcase-like device weighing ten pounds, not unlike the portable radio transmitters that spies use in World War II movies. It had a "Sampler" switch with "Sample" and "Trial" settings, and a "Dosage Scale" with only two calibrations: "Low" and "High."

None of the above-mentioned treatments originated at McLean. Indeed, none originated in the United States, and McLean was, in the scheme of things, a cautious adopter of new therapies. But McLean doctors did claim to have invented a curious goulash of the newly available therapies, to which they assigned the name "total push." In two papers published in 1939, Kenneth Tillotson and Abraham Myerson (who had evinced such an interest in the upper-class predilection for schizophrenia) out-

---

*I interviewed a McLean aide who witnessed a mass ECT session at the Greystone Park Psychiatric Hospital in Morristown, New Jersey. "That was a vivid experience," he said. "I saw about one hundred patients getting shock therapy in a huge room. They were all strapped down, and they were all twitching and jerking. This is the way they did it. I could just feel the electricity going through the air. There was no screaming, no physical agony, just this twitching."

lined an ambitious mobilization program that they adopted for a group of thirty-three McLean patients. They chose some of the stupefied, chronic "back-ward" types, "who sit on benches, stand in a corner or pace automatically to and fro, grimacing, passive and absorbed in [their] delusions," and decided to throw the book at them. Everything medical psychiatry had to offer was brought to bear on the target population: Nurses rousted them out of bed in the morning and forced them to go out on walks. Daily visits to the hydriatic suite for "showers, douches, massage and rubdowns" were de rigueur. Sports and athletics were empha-sized, and the patients received better food. But meals were no longer available through room service; total push forced the pa-tients to show up in the ward dining rooms to be fed. Patients who had been reluctant to eat were given a drug to stimulate their appetites. Vitamins were prescribed. The doctors forced men and women who had hovered around their wards in tattered bathrobes to dress neatly and present themselves to the general population. "Proper conduct" was reinforced with the granting of privileges, like access to "candy, ice cream . . . delicacies, cigarettes, and ci-gars," which were likewise withheld from malingerers. In his total push manifesto, Myerson seemed to be anticipating the future vogue of behaviorist psychology: "It would be interesting, but en-tirely impossible, to see what the effect of physical reward and physical pain would be, but society has not yet developed to the point where certain privileges and physical punishment can safely be used." Beating up on the Brahmin clientele was hardly McLean's style.

The psychological mobilization worked, supposedly, in tandem with the physiological shock therapies to get the dulled patients going again. (For some reason, Myerson also recommended the ultraviolet irradiation of the male patients' testicles, although he freely admitted that this procedure was "not related insofar as we know at present to the general well-being of the individual.") Not surprisingly, Tillotson declared total push to be a success. Of twenty-two patients he examined, he claimed that all had either slightly, much, or markedly improved. There was no later follow-up study because the outbreak of World War II effectively ended the total push experiment. McLean's luxurious 2:1 patient-to-staff ratio vanished into the wartime draft. A small army of male aides, nurses, and doctors left Belmont, and the staff-intensive total push experiment fell by the wayside.

∞

In our own time, it is not so unusual for men and women to discuss their stays in mental hospitals. Although most former patients still feel stigmatized by society at large, they know they are far from alone in their travails. From the high culture of literary memoirs to the low culture of talk shows, tales of life in the "bin" or the "zoo" are part of our cultural landscape.

But things were different in 1943, when a Boston businessman named Frank Kimball insisted on publishing the affecting story of his eleven-year stay at McLean. A trustee of Boston University, a churchgoer, and successful insurance and investment counselor, Kimball suffered a breakdown during his summer vacation in 1927. By his own account, he had become overwhelmed by his duties on his town's planning board and by the press of business. In December 1931 he transferred from the Channing Sanitarium in Wellesley, Massachusetts, to McLean.

Kimball promptly fell into what Abraham Myerson called the "prison stupor" that results when the shock of hospitalization interacts with the instinctual social retreat of the mental patient. Kimball described a "life of semi-automatic activity, in a blue fog of futility." His family rarely visited him: "What use was it for anyone to see me, when I sat like a wooden Indian? My handshake was cold, my greetings hardly more than dull murmurings."

In addition to his depressed state, he started to hear voices, a symptom of deepening schizophrenia.

One day my nurse happened to move a chair in my room, making a scraping noise. This sounded to me just as if he had said, gruffly, "Get out of here."

"What do you mean, telling me to 'get out of here'?" I complained.

"What? I never did."

Six years into his stay, the doctors started to "push" Kimball into activity. The patient librarian had launched a bimonthly magazine, *The McLean Gazette,* and asked him to contribute book reviews. He did, and he enjoyed doing it; however, he never spoke with the librarian, choosing to communicate with her only through handwritten notes. Then, in 1942, his doctors recommended electroshock therapy. Although none of the shock regimens turned out to "cure" or even significantly alleviate chronic schizophrenia, they had proved useful in combating depression. Kimball thought it was worth a try: "I don't remember much about it except for a dim recollection of trips in bathrobe and pajamas by wheelchair to the treatment room. There was little discomfort. I would be given the mild shock about 10:30 A.M., carried back to my room, and the first thing I knew I would awaken around noon, very much refreshed."

After three months of treatment, Kimball was encouraged to telephone his wife, Edith.

Edith was called to the phone.

"Hello," said the voice. "This is Frank."

"Who?"

"Frank."

"Frank who?" Edith was thinking of the boy who came to do odd jobs.

The voice, insistently. "It's Frank, your husband."

Edith was flabbergasted; she had not heard my voice on the phone for over fifteen years.

Kimball went back home to the Boston suburb of Dedham. He

returned to his church, he returned to his favorite hobbies—playing the piano and writing letters to the newspapers—and he was invited to rejoin Boston University's board of trustees. He served as toastmaster for his college class's fiftieth reunion, he flew in an airplane for the first time, and he even revisited McLean, accompanying his daughter-in-law in a musical revue. He had been saved, and he freely admitted he was not sure how or why:

"How can you *bear* to write so freely about all those bad years?" ask many of my friends. I have to smile. It has been a deep satisfaction right through—not a wink of sleep lost, not a twitch of a nerve from start to finish. Why, that old sourpuss in the story isn't me anyway! Perhaps never was. I don't know—I leave it to the psychiatrists to explain.

Lobotomies posed a classic clinical dilemma to the genteel, Harvard-trained McLean doctors. By the late 1930s, the controversial procedure had attained a certain legitimacy. The Portuguese doctor António Egasmoniz had first invaded a patient's frontal lobe in 1935, acting on the theory that destruction of the nerve connections behind the forehead broke up the "fixed ideas" that tormented schizophrenics. Almost immediately after reporting success in his first "leucotomies," Egasmoniz was nominated for a Nobel Prize, which he won in 1949. (Leucotomy, from the Greek word for "white," refers to the white fibrous material that Egasmoniz scraped from the front of the brain.) A brilliant and ambitious American doctor, Walter Freeman, seized on the Egasmoniz procedure and started performing "lobotomies" in Washington, D.C., in 1936. (Neither Freeman nor Egasmoniz was a surgeon, much less a neurosurgeon, a fact that did not escape their colleagues' notice.) Freeman and his surgical partner, James Watts, removed more of the frontal lobe than had Egasmoniz, hence the new nomenclature. They did not subscribe to Egasmoniz's theory that psychosurgery broke up fixed ideas in the patient's brain. Instead, they argued that lobotomy succeeded in severing contact between the frontal, "thinking" brain and the anterior, "feeling" part.

The results of the early lobotomies, indeed of all lobotomies, would prove to be equivocal. Eight of Freeman's first twenty patients had to have second operations. The postoperative reports tended to be vague, and soon enough grisly accounts of scalpel fragments breaking off inside patients' skulls began to surface. In promoting the procedure, science was the first casualty. Queried at a Boston psychiatric conference as to which kinds of patients were suited for lobotomy, Freeman answered, "The more this procedure is being used, the more indications there are for it."

Freeman, who eventually collaborated on more than a thousand lobotomies, was convinced he had struck the psychiatric El Dorado. The doctor in him knew he should be cautious in reporting successes, but Freeman the promoter was unable to restrain his enthusiasms, especially when a reporter's notebook or tape recorder happened to be nearby. "This woman went back home and in ten days she is cured," Freeman said of his first patient, a sixty-three-year-old woman from Topeka, Kansas. The woman resisted the surgery when she learned that her hair would have to be cut; Freeman promised her that he would do all he could to save her lovely curls. After the operation, he noted sardonically, "she no longer cared." His Norman Rockwell–like motto was "Lobotomy gets them home."

The media eagerly beat the drum for Freeman's "surgery of the soul," psychiatry's latest silver-bullet cure. "Surgery Used on the Soul-Sick," read the *New York Times* headline; "Relief of Obsessions Is Reported." In smaller type, the newspaper added that "new brain technique is said to have aided 65% of the mentally ill persons on whom it was tried as a last resort, but some leading neurologists are highly skeptical of it." Similarly enthusiastic reports appeared across the nation in magazines and local newspapers. The lobotomy vogue "hit us like a bomb," one American neurosurgeon recalled. By 1949, doctors were operating on 5,000 patients each year. Some leading neurologists were in fact skeptical, but as a measure of last resort lobotomy had a certain appeal. Bluntly put, the Freeman-Watts procedure had indeed cleaned some "human salvage" out of the back wards of many hospitals. Why not at McLean?

McLean doctors like to say they never evinced much enthusiasm for lobotomies, and statistics back them up. Between 1938 and 1941, no more than two patients received the operation each year. At its peak, in 1947, fourteen patients—all women—out of a census of around two hundred were lobotomized. (Two-thirds of McLean's patients at the time were women, and their average length of stay was much longer than the men's. Nationwide, doctors lobotomized twice as many women as men.) That peak may be partially explained by the upgrading of McLean's surgical facilities. Patients no longer had to be driven under guard into downtown Boston for surgery at the Massachusetts General Hospital. Now surgeons were only too happy to avail themselves of McLean's refurbished operating room. "With surgical fees running as high as $600 an operation," writes medical historian Jack Pressman, "psychosurgery had become a lucrative side-specialty."

Pressman obtained access to the case files of all McLean's lobotomy patients to write his 1998 history, *Last Resort: Psychosurgery and the Limits of Medicine.* On the one hand, he accepted the prevailing wisdom, articulated by acting psychiatrist-in-chief Paul Howard at a 1950 staff conference, that lobotomies were indeed "a last resort" for those long-term patients who had already failed to respond to less radical treatments. Howard allowed that the surgery may "take away something from the personality" but felt that it also held out the hope of relieving a life of suffering. But Pressman could not help but note how effortlessly the lobotomy option slid into the psychiatrists' checklist of possible cures. Initially envisaged as an option for patients who had lingered in the wards for more than two and a half years, it soon came to be discussed much earlier in the treatment cycle. "After a preliminary period of observation, electric shock and or insulin shock should be tried," one doctor noted in the file of a new arrival. "However, the prognosis in either therapy with this patient is not good and she may become a candidate for lobotomy." Pressman concluded, "For patients whose combination of age, sex, diagnosis, and mental history placed them in the pool of possible candidates, the meter was ticking as to the eventuality of receiving a lobotomy—a race between improving enough to be discharged from the hospital and being brought before a staff conference at which they would be recommended for surgery." At one such staff conference, a McLean doctor let slip that "we usually do a lobotomy to quiet people down."

Here is a transcript of a 1945 staff conference concerning the advisability of lobotomy for a male patient. The doctors' names have been changed.

MURPHY: Do you think he should have a lobotomy, Arthur?

BURDETT: I think it would be interesting to speculate what we would expect it to accomplish. . . . There is no thinking it is going to make him any worse except it might make him incontinent of urine.

MURPHY: It might make him dead or have convulsions.

BURDETT: I don't think that is very much worse than his present situation. I favor lobotomy, not with great enthusiasm, but I still favor it.

MURPHY: Dr. Green, what do you say?

GREEN: I do not feel qualified to express an opinion.

SWADLEY: I don't know what lobotomy would accomplish. . . .

MADDOX: From what I have read about lobotomies, those done on patients with real inner drive are more successful so this man might benefit.

AVERBUCK: Seems to me the fundamental disorder is not changed and I am opposed unless there is some very urgent need for it. . . .

MURPHY: One argument against the lobotomy is that he does not have a decent personality to go back to. . . . [On the other hand,] if we do not do a lobotomy the chances are he will just go along on Bowditch in this same state for many years.

KELLOGG: All the data in this record is on the hopeless side, but I do not have any definite opinion. I am rather against it as the risks are too great and the results too small. I wonder if he could be kept from deteriorating so rapidly by total push means.

At the end of the conference, the doctors voted not to lobotomize the patient in question.

At a small, well-staffed hospital like McLean, the doctors knew most of the patients personally. So when a patient like "Sarah Worthington" was lucky enough to make dramatic strides with the help of a lobotomy, every doctor knew about it. Worthington, a housewife and mother in her midforties, had been admitted to McLean in 1947 following a suicide attempt. The initial diagnosis was neurotic depression. At the hospital, she became aggressive and paranoid and again tried to commit suicide. She was given electroshock therapy, which depressed her even more. Five years of intense psychotherapy "might or might not help," opined one doctor, for "there is nothing to go back to in her case." About ten months after checking in, Worthington was lobotomized.

Her improvement was dramatic. She appeared at a rare postoperative staff conference and displayed "pleasure and spark." "The patient seems to have derived a good deal of protection from the overwhelming accumulation of her depressive feelings," her doctor noted. "It seems justifiable to say that the lobotomy has given her a chance to solve these problems in a way which no previous therapy had succeeded in doing." Her IQ was measured at 134—higher than before her surgery—and she was soon discharged home. Worthington found a job demonstrating merchandise to women's clubs and was promoted to a supervisory job after several years. She continued to meet her doctor for weekly psychotherapy and wrote him a grateful note several years after her surgery:

> I have been wishing to write to you a note of appreciation, not a senti-
> mental gushing expression of gratitude but an honest expression of
> how I feel in regard to your work. . . . When I first came to the hospi-
> tal I was in a room with no doors, no outlets. My only companions
> were Fear and Hopelessness. It was grim. Gradually throughout all of
> this time you have made me see for myself that particular room
> (which actually seems to have been of my own choosing) has doors. I
> am the one who must open them. I myself.

Of course, the doctors drew heart from Worthington's recovery.
But the statistical analysis was less forgiving. Of the first eight
women operated on, seven were still in McLean five years after
the surgery. At the 1950 staff conference, Paul Howard noted that
about half of the sixty patients lobotomized by then had been discharged from the hospital but still needed varying levels of care.
Those remaining in the hospital showed some improvement.
When I interviewed Howard almost fifty years later, even the distant memory of lobotomies sent a chill up his spine. "It's a horrible thing to think of, someone reaching into your brain and
cutting it with a knife." He still remembered the approximate
range of outcomes. "Our statistics showed that one-third of the
patients got a little better—these were people who had been in the
hospital for three or four years and probably weren't going to get
out—one-third got much better and one-third remained un-
changed."

McLean's flirtation with lobotomies ended in 1954. The newly
appointed director, Dr. Alfred Stanton, had a strong psychothera-
peutic background and zero interest in psychosurgery. Also, antipsychotic drugs were becoming available to the psychiatric
profession. Perhaps more importantly, the operation was develop-
ing an unsavory reputation. The irrepressible Walter Freeman had
decided to become the Henry Ford of psychosurgery, and he was
barnstorming the country to promote his gruesome "ice-pick" lobotomies. Instead of using anesthesia, Freeman, sometimes operating alone in his office in downtown Washington, electroshocked

his patients into unconsciousness. Then he hammered an ice pick (initially from the Uline Ice Company; later he used a surgical tool) through the bone above the eye and more or less randomly wiped out frontal lobe tissue. At the 1950 staff conference, Howard related a "probably fictitious story" about patients visiting Freeman's office for electroshock and emerging with two black eyes resulting from an impromptu lobotomy. Given Freeman's increasingly erratic conduct, it is possible that the story was true.

But there is another reason that lobotomies ground to a halt at McLean: Virtually every patient who might qualify for a lobotomy had already received one. Eighty-five percent of the lobotomized patients were discharged within eighteen months of having the operation. The rest hung around, taking up the few remaining beds for chronic sufferers. By 1954, McLean was already trying to admit younger patients, who held out more hope of being cured. "The salvageable deadwood had been logged out," Jack Pressman explained at the end of his study of psychosurgery at the hospital.

∞

In a bizarre coda to McLean's history with lobotomies, Walter Freeman drove his specially outfitted Cortez camper-van onto the property in 1968 and parked it outside of Upham Memorial Hall, then a geriatric ward. Freeman had converted his van into a mobile record room and carried hundreds of his own case files with him. He had even mounted an X-ray viewer inside the Cortez; Freeman was on a cross-country tour, seeking out former patients for the purpose of monitoring their progress and updating his files. (He had stopped performing lobotomies the previous year.) "He came on a weekend, and he wanted to be let in and have access to our records," recalls Dr. Paul Dinsmore, who was running Upham at the time. "I told him he couldn't just show up there off hours, and expect us to open our files." Freeman drove off, and did not return.

Freeman died in 1972, at the age of seventy-six.

#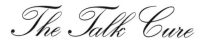

FREUD AND MAN AT MCLEAN

Great Doctor, are you savant or charlatan?
Abraham Bijur to Sigmund Freud

The Boston medical establishment, meaning the Harvard medical establishment, of which McLean was a part, did not leap to embrace Freudianism. This was somewhat ironic, given that Harvard doctors had played a key role in bringing Sigmund Freud's ideas to the United States. It was philosopher and psychologist (and putative McLean patient) William James who twigged onto Freud's work and discussed his ideas in his famous Gifford Lectures of 1901–1902, later published as *The Varieties of Religious Experience.* And McLean historian Silvia Sutton notes that Harvard neurologist James J. Putnam—the same Putnam who admitted Stanley McCormick to McLean—published the first paper in English on the clinical use of psychoanalysis in 1906 and "put Freud on the

American psychiatric map." Like many practitioners dipping their toes into the infant science of psychotherapy, Putnam's endorsement was tentative at best. His paper concluded "not that the 'psychoanalytic' method is useless, for I believe the contrary to be the case, but that it is difficult of application and often less necessary than one might think."

It was Putnam and Clark University president G. Stanley Hall who invited Freud, Jung, and Ernest Jones to Worcester, Massachusetts, to deliver a series of lectures at the university's twentieth-anniversary celebration in 1909. The event quickly acquired mythic proportions. Even the political agitator Emma Goldman, who had heard Freud speak in Vienna, attended the lectures; she had once operated an ice-cream parlor in Worcester with two anarchist colleagues. Freud himself called it "the first official recognition of psychoanalysis." It also proved to be Freud's only North American visit; to have appeared in the famous group photograph taken after the sessions was tantamount to immortality in the psychoanalytic pantheon. McLean was represented by F. Lyman Wells, a young assistant in pathological psychiatry, who told Hall he was entirely unimpressed. (James, too, was underwhelmed by Freud; "a man obsessed with fixed ideas," he reported.) Thomas Bond, a third-generation McLean psychiatrist, remembers his grandfather Earl telling him of his decision not to go to Worcester. "He thought Freud had no relevance to what they were doing at the asylum, and in a way he was right," his grandson said. Many McLean patients, then and now, were psychotically disturbed and deemed to be beyond the reach of Freud's intellectual "talk therapy."*

Freud's inroads into the psychiatric establishment came slowly. The first psychoanalyst hired by Harvard's Massachusetts General

---

*In 1928, Freud described his feelings about psychotic patients in a letter to Istvan Hollos: "I do not like these patients. . . . I am annoyed with them. . . . I feel them to be so far distant from me and from everything human. A curious sort of intolerance, which surely makes me unfit to be a psychiatrist."

Hospital, of which McLean was part, was stashed away in a cubby-hole under a flight of stairs, and his name was effaced, Soviet-style, from the hospital's official history. Starting in 1924, Freudian psychoanalysis begins to appear in the clinical section of McLean's annual report. In 1928, the director, Frederick Packard, wrote that "a special attempt has been made to find out what, if anything, in the Freudian methods is practical of application in the psychoses."

∞

Packard might have been entitled to his healthy skepticism over the usefulness of Freud's methods because just a few years before, he had admitted one of Freud's most famous patients, Dr. Horace Frink, into McLean. Frink occupies an unusual place in the history of psychotherapy; his was possibly the most famous disastrously botched analysis in the annals of Freudianism. A graduate of the Cornell Medical School, Frink pursued a brief surgical career before turning to psychiatry. Soon he became one of the first in a line of American ephebes who Freud hoped would proselytize his new science in the United States—"the most brilliant and promising of the young Americans," Freud called him. In 1911, Frink cofounded the New York Psychoanalytic Society with Abraham Brill and two other doctors, and he was unanimously elected its president in 1913. Five years later, Frink published a landmark study, *Morbid Fears and Compulsions;* forty years after its publication and twenty years after the author's death, Karl Menninger hailed it as "one of the clearest and best written expositions of psychodynamics." Not only was Frink smart, he was also a Gentile, which pleased Freud, who fretted constantly that psychoanalysis was attracting only Jews. An added plus was Frink's access to money via his attractive (married) mistress and patient, the comely Warburg family heiress Anjelika "Angie" Bijur, whom Freud encouraged the (married) Frink to wed.

When Horace Frink presented himself to Freud in person for the first time in the spring of 1921, he was in trouble. He had been experiencing occasional depressions for thirteen years and suffered from "toxic headaches," which could be relieved only by extended periods of relaxation. In Vienna, he was giddy, sleeping only a few hours a night and savoring the Austrian capital's heady nightlife in between his $10-an-hour sessions with "the master" in his office at 19 Berggasse. "I was very happy, and more talkative and full of fun than ever before in my life," Frink reported. Yet he also admitted to experiencing a "sense of unreality and an inability to form mental pictures."

A cynic, or a realist, might suggest that Frink's biggest problem was that he had started making love to his own patient, Madame Bijur. Aside from the obvious ethical concerns—Bijur had been his patient since 1912—there were complications. Horace's own wife Doris realized that he was unhappy in their marriage and was willing to grant him a divorce. But Anjelika's husband Abraham proved recalcitrant. Angie herself journeyed to Vienna in the spring of 1921, and Freud encouraged the two lovers to pursue their sexual destiny. As Madame Bijur later explained to the ubiquitous Adolf Meyer: "When I saw Freud, he advised my getting a divorce because of my own incomplete existence . . . and because if I threw Dr. F[rink] over now he would never again try to come back to normality and probably develop into a homosexual though in a highly disguised way."

Freud was alluding to Frink's purported unconscious homosexuality. Although Frink was alternately promiscuous and sexually equivocal—he once complained that Anjelika looked "queer, like a man, like a pig"—he is not known to have engaged in homosexual relationships.

In a letter to Anjelika's husband's analyst, Freud explained his conduct: "I simply read my patient's mind and so I found out that [Frink] loved Mrs. B., wanted her ardently and lacked the courage to confess it to himself. . . . I thought it the good right of every human being to strive for sexual gratification and tender love if he saw a way to attain them, both of which he had not found with his wife."

What ensued was worthy of a Georges Feydeau farce. Freud suggested that the two lovers confront the cuckolded husband, Abraham, in Paris and implore him to release his wife from her marital vows. All this came as a shock to Abraham, who thought his marriage might be saved. He had made love with Angie only a few days before and had just received a pair of $5,000 pearl studs from her as a token of her affection. Enraged, Mr. Bijur steamed back to New York and threatened a major scandal. He wrote Freud a long letter, which he intended to publish as a full-page advertisement in the New York press:

Dr. Freud:

Recently I am informed by the participants, two patients presented themselves to you, a man and a woman, and made it clear that on your judgment depended whether they had a right to marry one another or not. The man is at present married to another woman, and the father of two children by her, and bound in honor not to take advantage of his confidential position toward his patients and their immediate relatives. The woman he now wants to marry was his patient. He says you sanction his divorcing his wife and marrying his patient, but yet you have never seen the wife and learned to judge her feelings, interests and real wishes.

The woman, this man's patient, is my wife. . . . How can you know you are just to me; how can you give a judgment that ruins a man's home and happiness, without at least knowing the victim so as to see if he is worthy of the punishment?

. . . Great Doctor, are you savant or charlatan?

Luckily for Freud, Abraham died of cancer before he could publish the letter, which was forwarded to Vienna by Mr. Bijur's analyst. Freud responded tartly that the letter was silly and crafted to appeal to America's easily manipulated public opinion. But in fact, Freud was very worried about negative publicity, as he had every reason to be. In the 1920s, he was promoting psychoanalysis as a helpful, innovative new neuroscience, not a marriage-counseling service for anyone with a college education and boat fare to the Continent. Freud told Frink that he had specifically asked Anjelika not to "repeat to foreign people I had advised her to marry you on the threat of a nervous breakdown. It gives them a false idea of the kind of advice that is compatible with analysis and is very likely to be used against analysis." Freud, whose attraction to the American dollar was enhanced by Austria's rampant inflation, was also vulnerable to accusations of financial manipulation where the Bijur-Frink romance was concerned. Unbeknownst to him—at first—Angie had to settle $100,000 on Horace's first wife Doris to make her go away. Furthermore, Freud confirmed to his patient and disciple Frink that part of Mrs. Bijur's allure was her fortune:

> May I suggest to you that your idea Mrs. Bijur had lost part of her beauty may be turned into her having lost part of her money. If so I am sure she will recover her attraction. Your complaint that you cannot grasp your homosexuality implies that you are not yet aware of your phantasy of making me a rich man. If matters turn out all right let us change the imaginary gift into a real contribution to the psychoanalytic fund.

Dr. Silas Warner, who wrote a scholarly article on the "therapeutic disaster" that was the Freud-Frink relationship, notes that "the question has to be raised whether it was not Freud's fantasy that he would become a rich man from Mrs. Bijur's becoming Mrs. Frink, and making a substantial contribution to 'the psychoanalytic fund.'"

The therapeutic disaster begat a romantic disaster. Horace Frink and Anjelika Bijur did marry, but what Dr. Freud had joined together, it turned out, could easily be put asunder. With Freud having declared his analysis complete, Frink returned to the United States, where his depression and anxieties continued to haunt him.

He and Bijur lived separately, and each consulted Adolf Meyer. The Swiss-born Meyer was cooling on Freud's methods, and the Frink-Bijur mess sent him into the deep freeze. He called the case "nauseating." In 1924, when Angie's lawyer told Meyer that his client had "decided to obtain her freedom" from Dr. Frink, Meyer reacted furiously. Angie had seized upon Freud's suggestion of Frink's latent homosexuality, Meyer thought, when in fact Frink was simply the victim of a domineering wife. He fired back an answer to Bijur's lawyer: "Mere Freudian love-philosophy cannot guarantee safety and success in life as whole. Man is too complex a subject for that."

As Bijur proceeded with her divorce plans—this time from Frink—her husband became suicidal. He took an overdose of the barbiturates Veronal and Luminal, which his wife interpreted as a ploy to win back her affection. If so, it failed. She continued to plan their trip back to Paris for the purpose of annulling their French marriage. Ten days later, just before their ship was to sail, Frink deliberately cut the ulnar artery in the bend of his elbow. "The blood spurting out made an astonishingly loud noise," he reported, and it woke the male nurse sleeping in the room with him. Luckily, Frink was boarding with his old friend, Dr. Swepson Brooks, whose prompt intervention saved his life. Brooks and Bijur decided to commit Frink to McLean.

Shortly after Frink's arrival, Superintendent Frederick Packard—the man who would express a healthy skepticism concerning Freud's methods a few years later—wrote to Meyer that Frink's condition seemed to be improving. Frink had been doing some thinking, as well:

> He is very bitter against Freud, he says that Freud does not understand psychoses, that the field of psychoanalysis is limited to psychoneuroses, that Freud himself knew this and never should have attempted to treat him when he was in a psychotic condition and that his treatment and advice was all harmful and detrimental to his best interests.

Frink stayed at McLean for about five months and recovered nicely. He appeared at his own divorce proceedings after his release in 1925. He moved first to upstate New York and then to Chapel Hill, North Carolina, supporting his two children with money provided by his divorce decree and income from the few patients that he saw. "From the time of his release [from McLean] in April 1925 until a week before his death in 1936, he served as single parent to my brother John and myself, during which time he had no manic episodes," his daughter Helen wrote me. Suddenly, after eleven years of mental health, Horace Frink relapsed into catastrophic nostalgia for his bygone years. Reminiscing with his daughter over a watercolor of the Paris Opera House, he was assailed by the memory of his heady days with Anjelika Bijur. "Angie was radiant in a velvet cloak," he told Helen. "We stood looking over Paris. She turned to me and said, 'Horace, with your brains and my money, we can have the world.'" The next day he checked himself into Pine Bluffs Sanitarium in Southern Pines, North Carolina, and a week later he was dead of heart disease at age fifty-three. A packet of love letters was found next to his bed. No psychiatrist would dare say it, but Horace Frink had died of a broken heart.

Not long before his death, Helen asked her father what message she should give to Sigmund Freud, if she ever met him. Frink's answer: "Tell him he was a great man even if he did invent psychoanalysis."

Another well-known Freud analysand who became a familiar face at McLean was the editor, poet, and art collector Scofield Thayer.

Almost unknown today, Thayer was a brilliant, well-born literary and artistic entrepreneur who took over the editorship of *The Dial* during the brief period, from 1920 to 1925, when it could claim to be America's preeminent literary magazine. Thayer's *Dial* traced its roots to *The Dial* edited first by Margaret Fuller and then by Ralph Waldo Emerson in the 1840s, and it had become a money-losing, socialist soapbox for the likes of John Dewey, Charles Beard, and Thorstein Veblen when Thayer and his equally wealthy friend James Sibley Watson bought the magazine. Thayer and Watson turned *The Dial* into a money-losing, literary and artistic soapbox for the emerging expatriate avant-garde. Watson and Thayer poured thousands of dollars into the tiny (circulation 25,000) magazine, which was printed on paper good enough for reproducing works of art in full color. The owner-editors commissioned art from Oskar Kokoschka, Paul Signac, Pierre Bonnard, Henri Matisse, and Marc Chagall, and they published forty originals by Pablo Picasso. By the ripe old age of thirty-five, Thayer could claim to have known every major literary figure in America and Europe and to have published most of them. He was a close friend of T.S. Eliot, Thomas Mann, Ezra Pound, F. Scott Fitzgerald, and John Dos Passos, many of whom first reached an American audience in the pages of *The Dial*. Among its notable coups were the first U.S. publication of Eliot's *The Waste Land* and Mann's *Death in Venice*.

Poetically handsome ("strikingly pale, with coal-black hair, black eyes veiled and flashing, and lips that curved like those of Lord Byron" is *Dial* editor Alyse Gregory's overheated description of her employer and sometime love interest) and properly prepared at Milton Academy, Harvard, and Magdalen College, Oxford, Thayer was "too wealthy to have to work for a living and too interested in the arts to want to increase his inheritance by engaging in business," according to one chronicler. The Thayers were prominent in Worcester, Massachusetts, a thriving mill city at the turn of the century. Scofield's father owned several textile factories; his uncle Edward was nationally famous for his composition "Casey at the Bat." Thayer even had the right enemies; Gertrude Stein hated him for refusing to publish her poetry. He was an intimate and early promoter of E.E. Cummings, who penned a classical "Epithalamion" for Scofield's wedding to Elaine Eliot Orr and who later fathered a child with Elaine, apparently with Thayer's encouragement.*

As a youth, Thayer suffered from an unspecified nervous disorder and visited the eminent Manhattan psychotherapist Pierce Clark between twenty and thirty times a month. Like Horace Frink, Thayer had the resources and the will to travel to The Source. In 1920, he confided to his partner Watson that he hoped to travel to Vienna and become a patient of Freud's: "I am extremely eager to lay before him my troubles." After an exchange of letters, Freud accepted him as a patient the following year:

---

*The Elaine Orr Thayer–E.E. Cummings love-affair-turned-marriage-disaster is one of the great soap-opera love stories of the twentieth century. Scofield lost interest in his beautiful bride within fifteen months of their honeymoon. When they returned to New York, he took up residence in the Benedick, a luxury apartment building for bachelors, and she moved into Washington Square in Greenwich Village. Thayer encouraged Cummings to frequent Elaine and even reimbursed the penurious young poet for expenses incurred while entertaining his wife. The two became lovers, and Elaine became pregnant. Her daughter was born Nancy Thayer but was legally adopted by Cummings when he and Elaine married a few years later.

When Nancy was a young girl, her mother left Cummings for a man she fell in love with during a transatlantic crossing. Cummings was devastated, especially when Elaine insisted that their marriage be annulled to satisfy her new Catholic husband. As a result, Nancy was to know neither of her fathers. Her mother initially told her that Scofield was dead. When Nancy attained her majority, Elaine told her that Scofield was alive but insane. "But you needn't worry," Elaine said to Nancy, "it is not hereditary." The lawyer handling Scofield's affairs refused to let her visit the man she thought was her father "because you are said to resemble your mother."

Several years later, Nancy's mother let slip that she had once been married to Cummings, who had become one of the country's best-known poets. As if by coincidence, Cummings invited Nancy to visit him and his wife Marion at their farm in New Hampshire. Nancy found him charming and intelligent and allowed herself to wonder how her mother could have broken off relations with this wonderful man. At one point, while sitting for a portrait for Cummings, she thought, "I am falling in love with this man." Married with two children, Thayer decided to stop seeing the fifty-four-year-old poet. At their final interview, Cummings said, "Did anyone ever tell you I was your father?" The two remained friends until Cummings's death. Elaine Orr never warmed to the father-and-child reunion. She refused to discuss the paternity question with her daughter: "It was *my* life, and has nothing whatever to do with you," she said, adding, "your children will blame you for what you have done."

As a result of Cummings's disclosure, Nancy came into an unexpected inheritance. Although she had no claim on Scofield Thayer's vast art collection, conservatively valued at $10 million when he died, she became the executor of the Cummings estate after her father's death. And she assisted Richard S. Kennedy with his 1980 biography of Cummings, *Dreams in the Mirror*, from which this account is taken.

I am sorry I cannot get you fresh, your having gone through a long, unsuccessful treatment with another man is surely no advantage; yet let us hope that the incompetency of the analyst was for something in the matter, and that I will be able to justify your expectations. . . . Let me say in concluding that I feel very sympathetic about the determination you express to get out of your inhibitions or whatever it may be. The man who suffers deeply has a good chance to recover by analysis.

For a writer, Thayer left very little record of the time he spent with Freud. At times, when the analysis was going well, he talked of remaining in Vienna "indefinitely." At times it proceeded poorly. In a letter to his friend Alyse Gregory, Thayer wrote,

Speaking of the doctor [she had mentioned Freud] I might mention that he and I thanks to our "good" recent dreams and rather agreeable recent remarks of his own are to each other somewhat reconciled. We talked things over from the practical point of view yesterday and he now gives on record his feeling that we are making some advances and is hoping that in time we may get somewhere.

Thayer's life in Vienna clearly revolved around Freud. In one letter, he recounted bringing a Chagall watercolor he was thinking of buying to Freud for his approval, which was granted. Eighteen months into his analysis, like a bolt from the blue, Thayer announced that Freud has agreed to write for *The Dial:* "I have obtained from Freud an article," he wrote to New York editor Kenneth Burke, "about 30 pages in length, elucidating a church account of the selling of a man's soul to the devil in Austria in the 17th century. I consider this a scoop. As in all Freud's writings, so here also, there are, of course, passages in which 'details' are mentioned."

Thayer was talking about sexually explicit details, and he left it to his New York–based colleague to determine whether Freud's work was suited for the Yankee audience. Whatever they decided,

"Freud absolutely refuses to have anything cut or to have any passage in any way altered. . . . Professor Freud is willing to have certain words (penis, etc.) translated as non-grossly as possible, but is not willing to make any further concessions whatsoever."

Not for the first time, Freud had cut himself a good deal. Thayer agreed to pay Freud the unusually high fee of two cents a word if the article was accepted. Thayer was paying for what we today would call third serial rights; Freud had already sold the same article to the German magazine *Imago* and to the *International Psycho-Analytic Journal.* If *The Dial* rushed the piece into print, they would beat out the *Journal* by a month, hence Scofield's "scoop." For reasons unknown, *The Dial*'s New York editors rejected the article.

Thayer remained in Vienna for more than two years, savoring the cultural high life. He befriended the writer Arthur Schnitzler and seemed to spend almost every evening at the opera or symphony and added to his astonishing art collection. It is unclear why he ended his analysis, and even his comments on Freud are maddeningly inconsistent. "When I leave Vienna, I shall, after two years forced compression, be chock full of the Great Man," he wrote to Gregory, his lifelong friend with whom he constantly flirted in his letters. (After his analysis, he tried to lure her to Europe to spend the summer with him, "having in view the possibility of surveying the Unconscious.") Thayer knew that his slavish deference to Freud muddled his own efforts at self-understanding. "I follow Freud's gestures seeking dreams as does a dog who, when his master throws, leaps forward and away for the stone," he wrote in a note to himself. "And in this case (as often with the dog) one does not know but that the hand was empty."

Thayer started to break down in the summer of 1925, which he spent at his Edgartown home on Martha's Vineyard. He was cultivating a bizarre feud with Philadelphia's renowned art collector Dr. Albert Barnes, who was competing with Scofield for the masterpieces flowing from the brushes of Picasso, Georges Braque, Matisse, and Fernand Léger. Thayer asked his friend Watson to send him a gun from New York so he could defend himself from his "enemies."* Although he clearly had doubts about his experiences with Freud, whom he privately derided as a "privateer," he was also angling to become a patient again. But it was not to be. Freud's worries about the recurrence of his cancer caused him to cut his patient roster down to just six. Thayer offered to buy out another patient's slot, but Freud would not hear of it. A few months later, Scofield resigned as editor of *The Dial* and took up residence at Upham Memorial Hall on the grounds of McLean.

Thayer stayed at McLean twice but became better known as an occasional visitor. He was so rich that he did not need to stay in a mental hospital or sanitarium for very long. For almost sixty years Thayer and his two male nurses became familiar figures at Butler Hospital in Worcester, at the Craig House sanitarium in Beacon, New York, as well as the St. Regis and Biltmore hotels in New York City, the Hotel Beau Rivage at Ouchy-Lausanne (where Stanley and Katharine McCormick had their wedding reception), or the Grand in Venice. McLean doctors remember Thayer dropping by Proctor Hall, one the hospital's geriatric units, for occasional work-ups and suggestions of new approaches for dealing with his dementia. After a consultation involving a promising new drug or the therapeutic regimen of the moment, the trio would disappear back to Florida or to Edgartown or to a luxury hotel.

By way of life commentary, Thayer left thousands of short, undated notes narrating virtually all aspects of his life. They are articulate and occasionally insightful but suffused with the terrible random anger that presumably dragged Thayer's "normal" behavior into madness. He wrote detailed descriptions of his wife's sex organs and devoted several hundred scraps of paper to what reads like a homoerotic fixation on a friend in Bermuda. In one notebook, he jotted down the following entries, in order:

---

*Watson was armorer to the stars. He provided E.E. Cummings with a 38-caliber pistol during the dramatic breakup of the Thayer-Cummings marriage. Cummings was threatening a murder-suicide scenario that, happily, never took place.

He who has known masturbation can never be satisfied with marriage.

When the penis enter the vagina—note the position of said vagina—to the girl it's all dark meat.

Publish edited Gibbon.

The Latin ablative absolute is alone worth the whole Greek language.

When Thayer died in 1982, neither the *New York Times* nor the *Boston Globe* published an obituary of the man who had shepherded so many crucial European and American artists and writers into the literary canon. For public consumption, Thayer had been out of circulation since 1926. An only child whose daughter Nancy had been legally adopted by Cummings, he had no living relatives at the time of his death. His fabulous art collection went to New York's Metropolitan Museum—a stinging blow to the Worcester Art Museum, where it had "temporarily" resided for almost fifty years. (Thayer's will dated back to the 1920s, when the relative positions of the Worcester and New York museums were not so disparate as in 1982.) His writing, letters, and notes ended up at Yale's Beinecke Rare Book Library, where I found this tiny, penciled memorandum among his effects:

> *I have not loved the world*
> *Nor the world me.*

∽

Until the late 1960s, McLean had a celebrity patient named Carl Liebman. Unlike other celebrity patients such as Robert Lowell or Ray Charles, Liebman was a psychiatric celebrity. Over the span of a half-century, he had been attended by almost every major figure in European and American psychiatry—Sigmund Freud, Otto Rank, Eugen Bleuler, Ruth Mack Brunswick, Manfred Sakel, Abraham Brill—and received every form of treatment known to *homo psychiatricus:* psychoanalysis, insulin shock, electroshock, hydro-therapy, and a topectomy—a sort of minilobotomy. In the 1960s, Liebman developed a small following at McLean because he was one of the few surviving analysands from Freud's Vienna years. Young residents concocted pretexts to drift by Upham Memorial, the lavishly appointed "Harvard Club," where Liebman spent his waning years. Tall, gaunt, intermittently erudite and noncommunicative, he was a genuine museum piece, as close as many of the young trainees would ever come to the headwaters of Continental psychoanalysis. "I knew him on Upham, and he used to talk about his time with Freud, and how they would argue about philosophers and so forth," says Dr. Harold Williams. "The lobotomy didn't interfere with his thinking processes; it was visible, but it wasn't one of those ice-pick jobs." It goes without saying that Liebman's case file, with original letters from Freud and a catalogue raisonné of therapeutic gambits, was required reading for historically minded young doctors. (Indeed, it was after several original letters from Freud went missing from Liebman's file in the mid-1960s that McLean restricted staffers' access to its record room.) Longtime McLean neuropathologist Dr. Alfred Pope remembers the date of Liebman's death in 1969 quite precisely because Pope was among those who were hoping for a clinical pathology conference on the deceased patient. In the end, there was neither a conference nor an autopsy. Pope in particular had been hoping to get (another) piece of Liebman's brain for his experiments on the chemical architecture of the schizophrenic cortex. He had managed to scrounge some cerebral tissue from Liebman's 1950 topectomy at the hospital. "It was kind of a bonanza," he recalled. A postmortem tissue sample would have added to the coup. Liebman's brain was arguably the most worked-over cerebral cortex in psychiatric history. The details of Liebman's treatment still bring a bemused smile to Harold Williams's face. "Here's a guy who suffered through all the horrible stuff psychiatry could throw at him, and still managed to survive."

Born at the turn of the century, Liebman was the only son of a wealthy New York beer magnate, Julius Liebman, one of the Brooklyn-based brewers of the Rheingold label. "His personality was always, already as a boy, different from that of most children," according to his Park Avenue physician Dr. Leopold Stieglitz, who added: "He did not readily take part in sports and athletic exercises, was if anything, afraid of doing things such as climbing trees. His mother at times tried to overcome this disinclination on his part by twitting him and then the boy would give in rather reluctantly."

In 1918, Carl Liebman went off to Yale, where he ran track, was a private in the precursor of the Reserve Officers' Training Corps, and lived in a single room for three out of four years. Stieglitz reported that his New Haven stay was not a happy one. "He was called a 'fairy' by the boys and acknowledged to me that he enjoyed seeing the nude bodies of the boys in the swimming pool and occasionally had dreams of an erotic nature in connection with these boys," he wrote. "He particularly enjoyed wearing a jock strap and seeing the boys when they wore a jock strap." In later analyses, Liebman would report that he experienced sexual excitement at the sight of a jockstrap as early as age twelve. During adolescence, he developed obsessional fears about the safety of his sperm, which he called "spermanimalcules," worrying that by ejaculating them, he was committing genocide. After Liebman graduated, Stieglitz referred him to his Upper East Side colleague, Dr. Pierce Clark–Scofield Thayer's doctor–who contributed a preliminary diagnosis of fetishism. Clark proved to be the first stop in Carl Liebman's Grand Tour of world psychiatry.

After a brief analysis with Clark, Liebman took off for Europe, supposedly to pursue his career as an artist. In Zurich, he quickly came under the influence of Oskar Pfister, a Swiss Protestant minister, lay analyst, and close friend of Freud. Pfister in turn handed him off to Dr. Eugen Bleuler, head of Zurich's prestigious Burgholzli Psychiatric Clinic and a celebrity headshrinker favored by transatlantic Yanks. ("A great imbecile," his patient Zelda

Fitzgerald called him.) Bleuler spent forty-five minutes with Lieb-man in 1924, during which time the patient fidgeted constantly and showed early signs of what would later become deep compulsions. Liebman talked about his urge to constantly wash his hands and his fears of the way people seemed to stare at him on the street. "It was *how* he talked about this that seemed schizophrenic," Bleuler reported. From Pfister and Bleuler, Liebman moved on to the Big Show: Sigmund Freud accepted him as a patient in 1925.

"Do not worry about your young American," Freud wrote to Pfister, "the man can be helped." Freud met with Liebman's parents, Julius and Marie, and fretted about their role in their son's analysis: "They seem very willing to make sacrifices, which generally points to a bad prognosis." The analysis itself proceeded in fits and starts. In August 1925, Freud wrote to Pfister, "As for your young hopeful, I think you should let him go to his ruin." But just two months later, he changed his mind. "I began feeling sorry for the poor lad," he wrote to Pfister. "I had a change of heart." Freud confided to the parents that there were two good reasons for not continuing his sessions with their son. For one thing, Carl needed years of work, and Freud, who feared he was experiencing a recurrence of his oral cancer, worried that he might not live to finish the case. Also, he was concerned that Liebman's condition might worsen. "My third and last motive, that I wanted to spare myself a terrible amount of trouble, I kept to myself," Freud wrote.

Freud continued to see Carl Liebman for five more years while his patient was pursuing graduate work at the University of Vienna. He chronicled his relationship with the wealthy young American in letters to Pfister:

> With our lad . . . things are going very strangely. . . . I was again very near the point of giving him up, but there is something touching about him which deters me from doing so; the threat of breaking off the treatment has made him gentle and amenable again, with the re-

sult that at present a good understanding prevails between us. . . . What weighs on me in his case is my belief that, unless the outcome is very good indeed, it will be very bad indeed; what I mean is that he would commit suicide without any hesitation. (January 3, 1926)

Tomorrow I am sending [Liebman], who has been here since August 1, on holiday until October 1. I must tell you about him, there have been many changes in his case. His intolerableness has been successfully overcome, I have actually grown fond of him, and he seems to reciprocate this. After dreadful difficulties, some pieces of the secret history of his development have been laid bare, and the effect, as was corroborated by relatives who saw him during the holidays, has been very favorable. . . . On the other hand it is undeniable that there is a great deal about him that is alarming, as if he were on the way to passing from obsessional neurosis to paranoia. . . . I propose to leave aside the academic question of diagnosis and go on working with the living material. (September 14, 1926)

[Liebman] has not yet given up his childish reactions to the influence of authority, and it is that that makes him so difficult to treat. I am not wasting time on the question of correct diagnosis; he certainly has plenty of schizophrenic traits. . . . the lad is a severe ordeal. I am trying hard to get him to deliberately resist his fetishistic masturbation to enable him to corroborate for himself all that I have discerned about the nature of the fetish, but he will not believe that such abstinence will lead to this and is essential for the progress of the treatment. On the other hand I feel a great deal of sympathy for him, and cannot make up my mind to send him away and risk a disastrous outcome. (April 11, 1927)

In 1928, in a letter to Marie Liebman, Freud ventured a diagnosis: "I have no right to keep from you that the diagnosis in your son's case is Paranoid Schizophrenia." He admitted that "such a diagnosis means little and does not help penetrate the uncertainty about his future. Even [Jean-Jacques] Rousseau was such a case, not less abnormal. Whenever I examine the analysis I tell myself that one couldn't do anything for him but to give him much out of which he *himself* can make something." Marie would later remark that her son understood that Freud had given him permission to embark on a "self-analysis," which in his case meant holing up in a hotel room and shunning the outside world. In 1930, Freud gave up on Liebman and shunted him off to his own analysand and "adoptive daughter," the American Ruth Mack Brunswick, apparently hoping that a female analyst might help Carl overcome his sexual fetishes. According to psychiatrist David Lynn, who reviewed Liebman's case file at McLean, the patient got nowhere with Brunswick. He "withdrew into his psychosis, declared an end to his relations with his parents, and saw Freud one last time, in 1931."

By interviewing Liebman's doctors at McLean, Lynn culled many droll tidbits about the five-year-long, failed analysis. (Observing McLean guidelines, Lynn identified Liebman with the pseudonymic initials "A.B.") During his meetings with Freud, Liebman remembered the great doctor's chow dog seated quietly at his master's feet. Freud generally smoked a cigar, waving it in the air to punctuate his speech. (Other patients reported that Freud lit cigars to celebrate diagnostic insights.) Freud never offered Liebman a cigar, which the patient interpreted as a rejection of his manhood. In sum, a bad experience for all concerned.

Like Thayer and Frink, Liebman was not a successful patient of Dr. Freud. After his brief acquaintance with Dr. Brunswick, Liebman journeyed to Paris for a few sessions with the celebrated Dr. Otto Rank, who first hypothesized on "birth trauma." Soon afterwards he returned to New York City, traveling steerage and arriving with $150 in his pocket. He lived alone in the Mills Hotel and sent occasional postcards to his family. Seeking financial independence from his parents, he took driving lessons in order to become a cabdriver and washed cars at night to pay his way. But he soon ended up back in the parental ambit, accepting a small allowance from his father plus the use of a car. He started driving his father to and from the Brooklyn brewery, but he proved to be a less-than-ideal chauffeur. While driving, "he was possessed with the fear of running over a child" and continually looked back over his shoulder to see if he had hit anyone. In 1933, in his parents' bathroom, Liebman stripped to the waist and drove a bowie knife into his rib cage, beneath the left nipple. Even though the knife tip missed Carl's heart by just a half-inch, the phlegmatic family doctor Stieglitz characterized the "performance" as "rather theatrical," a classic suicide "gesture." Immediately afterwards, Liebman was sent to yet another distinguished analyst, the increasingly famous Abraham Brill. After Frink's breakdown, Brill had assumed the mantle of America's Number One Freudian; he was chief of the New York Psychoanalytic Society and translator of Freud's early works into English, Brill's second language. It was Brill who recommended what would prove to be a lifetime stay at McLean. Noting that Liebman had been seen by no fewer than six psychiatrists in his brief lifetime—Dr. Hermann Nunberg, a Viennese disciple of Freud who had emigrated to Philadelphia had been added to the mix—Brill concluded that "analysis gave [Liebman] considerable insight, but has not at all changed his delusional trend." As an example of such a delusion, Brill noted that Liebman "imagined that he was followed by detectives." In a letter written at almost the same time, Liebman's sister Kitty explained to McLean officials that the family knew of their son's various New York adventures because "we had him followed by detectives from the time he left Vienna. He knows nothing of this." It is true; even paranoids have enemies.

Upon admission to McLean, Liebman and his family joined in a ghoulish debate over whether he should reenter analysis inside the hospital. In 1935, McLean was pushing a precursor of milieu therapy, placing their patients in a salubrious, comfortable, non-threatening environment and hoping for the best. Carl wanted more psychoanalysis, but his mother argued no. "If Drs. Pfister, Freud, Ruth Mack Brunswick, Brill and Nunberg have not helped you by analysis, it is pretty well proven that analysis will not help you," she wrote to her son's McLean doctor. She added, "Freud had given him up, saying: 'I have given you all of which analysis is capable, now you must try to get along by yourself' (which I fear Carl Liebman has construed as his own written self analysis of which even Freud told him, I could not cure)."

But in a ten-page, handwritten cri de coeur addressed to his parents from the hospital, Liebman protested his forced incarceration ("a police arrest") and his inability to engage in "self-analysis," or any kind of analysis, at McLean:

> Practically, I am under constant surveillance. The door must be ajar, and always constantly there are people in the corridor. . . . In the morning I do a few exercises in the gym, then I go to the clay-modelling room, by way of occupational therapy. At 11 o'clock a shower with pulse-taking and other hokum under guard (with a nurse). I am permitted to walk about a dozen times around the yard. In the afternoon I am permitted to return to the pottery or play billiards with my usually amiable nurse. None of this is difficult; it is not even compulsory, but it is inane. It is what my doctors are pleased to call an ordered existence. I am living in a vacuum.

Psychiatrists who analyzed Liebman always mentioned his intelligence and his ability to articulate his dilemmas, even if he seemed incapable of solving them. In this first letter from McLean, Carl correctly predicted a long stay:

> I am here as long as the doctors "see fit." . . . My condition here will be a vicious circle. It will be continually worse. The doctors will not release me now and presumably they will not release me later—and not for many years. When I am released it will be too late and in addition the people in whose recognition of modest achievements I might have taken pleasure will be dead. Prof. Freud will be dead—perhaps you will be dead.

Almost immediately, Carl's father wrote back, explaining the family's motivation for the forced commitment.

Dear Carl,

You may not have appreciated our heartache and worry for you while you were home, but it was there all the time. We felt that in spite of trying to fit in with all your wishes your being at home did not keep you from becoming increasingly ill. You yourself often complained that you felt as if you were standing on your head and could not control yourself. You know as well as we that should you have lost control you would have been forced into a state institution where your chance of helpful medical treatment can not be compared with McLean. It was difficult for us to make this decision and we did not consult you because we knew that we could not get you to agree—since having had analysis for so many years—you did not believe in psychiatry.

Even the analysts Doctors Freud, Mack Brunswick, Brill and Nunberg felt that analysis could no longer help you, having tried it for over nine years, and the ones consulted here insisted it was only fair to give you medical treatment. Whatever you may think about us, we have considered your welfare above our own.

Carl contemptuously dismissed the McLean routine as "eggnogs, shower-baths and occupational 'therapy.'" But in fact, the hospital had many cures in mind for him. Within months of Liebman's arrival, Dr. Manfred Joshua Sakel passed through McLean and met with him, among others. Not surprisingly, Liebman's parents authorized Sakel to perform his innovative insulin coma therapy on Carl. There is no evidence that it accomplished much. Nurses' notes indicate that Liebman remained paranoid. Around Christmas time in 1935, a nurse took him shopping in nearby Waverley Square.

On going out into the street, patient kept walking around looking behind him. Stopping several times to look behind him and to stare into space. Patient on seeing anyone coming down the sidewalk would rush onto the pavement outside the parked cars, apparently to avoid meeting them. Mr. Liebman did not seem conscious of the traffic. . . . On returning after crossing the railroad tracks on which a train was approaching, patient suddenly stopped, turning quickly walked back toward the bars, saying "it seems good to see a train again."

Carl also attempted a feeble "escape" that year. He attacked a fellow patient in 1943. In 1948, he made a supervised visit to his parents in New York. The following year, psychiatry unveiled its latest panacea for Carl's suffering. Yet another doctor from New York's Upper East Side traipsed up to McLean in 1949 to examine the disturbed patient. As always with doctors, Liebman impressed him with his general articulateness and mastery of certain conversational subjects. "My recommendations that topectomy be performed rather than a lobotomy were based on the patient's apparent intellectual preservation and the desirability of maintaining as much intellectual function as possible," this doctor wrote. Liebman underwent a topectomy, performed by the man who had invented the procedure, in the operating room at McLean.

Just a year later, another New York doctor traveled northwards from Craig House, a pricey psychiatric sanitarium, to interview Carl. "I took the opportunity of asking him whether he considered his illness a neurosis or a psychosis and I used those words," Dr. Jonathan Slocum reported to McLean's superintendent Dr. Franklin Wood. "His answer was that he was not qualified to say, but that he believed that the diagnosis of 'Paranoid schizophrenia was probably correct.'" Slocum continued:

I am certain in my own mind that the one thing this man must not have is freedom. I believe firmly that his greatest unhappiness comes not from his being restricted, but from his conflict. I have not been asked for a recommendation, but I would say that he should go on as is and if he becomes unmanageable, that a deep lobotomy should be considered, because he possesses [sic] a great threat to those around him.

The radical lobotomy was never performed.

Carl Liebman's condition never improved. But he did become better known. Although the first analysts trained primarily in Freudian methods showed up at McLean in the late 1930s, it was not until the centennial of Freud's birth—1956, when his face appeared on the cover of *Time* magazine—that virtually every man and woman entering psychiatry were steeped in Freudian teachings. The New York and Boston Psychoanalytic Institutes, which certified "genuine" Freudian analysts, reigned supreme. The top spots in academic psychiatry were reserved for the men and few women who had undergone a multiyear training analysis with an Institute-certified doctor. Small wonder that Carl Liebman became a celebrity at McLean.

Liebman stories abound, such as his greeting doctors on the manicured pathways with the salutation "I am my father's penis." That greeting ended when one interlocutor countered with "Good morning, Mr. Penis." In his old age, Liebman had substituted a relatively common hand-washing fetish for the more exotic jockstrap fixation of his youth. "He thought he was tainted with a sexually transmitted disease, and if he could, he would get a hold of surgical tape and bind his hands," recalls Dr. Paul Dinsmore, who administered Upham while Liebman was there. "Then he would get contractions, which was a shame, because he was a talented artist. He could have had more privileges, but when he got off the grounds he would go down to Corbett's drugstore and get more surgical tape to bind his hands."

By the 1960s, Liebman was just another debilitated old man serving out his sentence at McLean. Nurse Constance Holian remembers him as unsociable but popular among the dotty Upham crowd. He was famous as the Man Who Knew Freud, but he was hardly an advertisement for the achievements of talk therapy: "We used to joke that Freud didn't do him much good," she recalls.

Welcome to the Twentieth Century

> Damn it Harry, schizophrenia is not all that tough.
> It should be easy to cure.
>
> **Alfred Stanton to Dr. Harry Sullivan**

*The McLean culture of relaxed, custodial care for mildly-to-very-*batty aristocrats reached a nadir in the immediate postwar years. Franklin Wood, the bow-tie-wearing Rotarian, ran the hospital on a cash-and-carry basis, relying on his tiny three-ring spiral note-book for guidance on all matters of policy, personnel, and patient care. Visiting the wards with a red carnation firmly planted in his lapel, Wood represented the end of an era. He would be the last nonpsychiatrist to run the hospital, and he would be the last director to occupy the stately superintendent's residence, where he stabled his family and a brace of pet Dalmatians, just down the hill from Eliot Chapel. Harvard had appointed Wood for his administrative skills; the clinical work was overseen by the psychiatrist-in-chief, Kenneth Tillotson. A bumptious, outgoing soul, Tillotson would later earn a footnote in literary history as the doctor whose electroshock therapy so traumatized Smith College junior Sylvia Plath that she attempted suicide shortly thereafter. But first Tillotson would gain wider renown, which unexpectedly transformed him and his hospital into the laughing-stocks of Boston.

Tillotson had a roving eye, and it landed on his subordinate, one Anne Marie Salot, a twenty-eight-year-old nurse who is described in Silvia Sutton's official history of McLean as "a very good looking brunette." Salot had had an affair with her boss, which, she claimed in a complaint to the State Department of Mental Health, had cost her her job. (Her complaint also stated that Tillotson's continuing interest in her was jeopardizing her mental health.) Not surprisingly, her charges cost Tillotson *his* job. The McLean trustees, hastily assembled in the downtown offices of "Mr. Boston," their chairman Ralph Lowell, gave Tillotson the heave-ho.

In time-honored Brahmin tradition, McLean managed to keep *l'affaire* Tillotson quiet. The resignation of the hospital's chief psychiatrist and his disappearance from the roster of the Harvard Medical School went unnoticed. The Boston Braves were in the World Series; the press had more important stories to cover. But then the state decided to pursue morals charges against the pair, and the media circus was on.

"Dr. K.J. Tillotson and Nurse Held on Morals Charge," the *Boston Sunday Globe* announced on November 2, 1948. The Boston papers salted their coverage with eloquent photos of the comely Ms. Salot and the staid Dr. Tillotson, whose mousy, bespectacled wife always accompanied him to the courtroom. (At one hearing, readers learned, "Miss Salot was clad in a white wool dress, tailored black coat and black hat with veil, and fashionable strapped black suede shoes." There is no offsetting description of Mrs.

Tillotson.) Tillotson was mischievously described as "a world famous psychiatrist" because he had once testified in Washington on behalf of *Esquire* magazine, which had started printing girlie pictures for its GI audience in 1942. In its quest to yank *Esquire*'s second-class mail permit, the post office found a psychiatrist to inveigh against the magazine. But Tillotson showed up to defend the "good clean pictures glorifying good figures and a tribute to American womanhood." Sutton writes, "That episode was resurrected from the depths into which it had supposedly sunk and was repeated again and again in newspaper articles as though it were evidence of Tillotson's lascivious nature." When the hullabaloo reached fever pitch, Tillotson and Salot quickly copped guilty pleas to dodge the limelight. Like a purged commissar, Tillotson, who had run McLean in the early 1930s and had served as psychiatrist-in-chief for fifteen years, saw his name vanish from the official histories of McLean and its parent, the Massachusetts General Hospital. Explains Sutton, "Officially, Tillotson had become persona non grata because he had committed the unpardonable sin of tarnishing McLean's respectability."

The press ridiculed McLean because a juicy sex story is a juicy sex story but also because the hospital was in a position to be ridiculed. Across the country, psychoanalysis and psychology, infant sciences in America between the wars, were gaining rapid acceptance after World War II. The Army trained a generation of psychiatrists to treat soldiers suffering from shell shock and other battlefield traumas, and once demobilized, these men fanned out across the country to bolster the reputations of the top sanitariums: the Menninger Clinic in Topeka, Kansas; Austen Riggs in Stockbridge, Massachusetts; or Hillside in New York. In Boston, the state-run Boston Psychopathic Hospital, later the Massachusetts Mental Health Center, had eclipsed McLean in reputation. Even the Veterans Administration hospitals were centers of innovation and creative thinking. But the rush of change had left Wood, Tillotson, and McLean in its wake. The hospital had become an undistinguished backwater.

A visiting psychiatrist who spent a summer at McLean in the 1950s reported that "the atmosphere is almost medievalistic or feudalistic." This visitor continued, "Pay is at a stinkingly low level because it is presumably offset by altruistic satisfactions and loyalty rewarded." Pay and money, as it happened, were very much on Franklin Wood's mind. In one of his annual reports, he complained that "the problem of money has become all important." A key factor in McLean's rising costs, he intimated, was the staff's vulgar desire to be compensated with lucre rather than with room, board, and paternalistic love. Some "employees of many years of faithful service behind them" still seemed to enjoy their work and do their jobs "because they feel they are doing their part to help others. Yet this group of people is becoming smaller every year," Wood wrote. Altruism was in increasingly short supply: "No longer does the feeling of satisfaction in a job well-done and the helping of others serve as a goal. Money seems to be the predominant aim of today."

Midcentury McLean "had a very mixed reputation," remembers Stephen Washburn, who grew up in nearby Newton, attended Harvard Medical School, and joined the hospital staff in the mid-1950s:

> I heard really wild stories about McLean, about people running across the campus in the nude, and then of course there was this story about Dr. Tillotson, and that was a disaster for the hospital. It had this kind of seedy reputation from Dr. Wood's day. There was not a lot going on except that people were being entertained.

McLean needed a savior, and they needed one fast.

∞

In 1955, the trustees decided to hire Alfred Stanton, a tall, cerebral New Jersey native who had recently moved to the Veterans Administration hospital in Boston. Stanton was brainy, moralistic—he was reared a Quaker, and even as an adult addressed his brother in "thees" and "thous"—and medically modern. Psychoanalytically trained, he was an intellectual disciple of Harry Stack Sullivan, a neo-Freudian who believed psychotherapy could be successfully applied to severely disturbed schizophrenics. At the Chestnut Lodge sanitarium in Rockville, Maryland, Stanton worked closely with Frieda Fromm-Reichmann, a prominent exponent of Sullivan's theory that mental illness stemmed not from childhood trauma but from damaged interpersonal relationships. Fromm-Reichmann was perhaps better known to a mass audience as the empathetic "Dr. Fried" who cures the troubled "Deborah Blau" in Hannah Green's best-selling autobiographical novel *I Never Promised You a Rose Garden.* Stanton himself makes a brief appearance in the book as the unfriendly "Dr. Royson," who takes over Deborah's case while Dr. Fried is on vacation. The author invokes the doctor's "austerity of manner" and "icy logic" and even assigns him a nickname: "Dr. Snake-tooth." (More disturbingly, she burns herself with a cigarette to protest the unwanted change of therapists.) Stanton, invariably described by colleagues as formal and stuffy, was nothing if not self-aware; he pointed out the unflattering passage to his elder son in a bookstore. "He didn't take offense at it," Bruce Stanton recalls. "He kind of chuckled and said it was his literary claim to fame."

Stanton had another, more imposing claim to literary fame. In hiring him, McLean had hired the man who wrote the book on the modern mental institution—literally. Just one year before he came to McLean, Stanton had published *The Mental Hospital,* coauthored with sociologist Morris Schwartz. (Schwartz would become famous to a different generation as the title character of the best-selling book *Tuesdays with Morrie.*) The two men had spent three years observing the complex relationships among doctors, nurses, staff aides, and patients on the disturbed ward of the Chestnut Lodge sanitarium in Rockville, Maryland. The result was the 492-page book, clearly written by the dense standards of psychoanalytic literature, which remained a standard text for budding psychiatrists well into the 1960s. One Boston doctor now in his sixties remembers his supervisor commenting upon a severe, ongoing disturbance on the locked ward of Massachusetts Mental Health Center with the words "Gentlemen! I give you Stanton and Schwartz."

Stanton's book—the profession regards the ideas as his, the writing as Schwartz's—advanced the idea, in fact, *proved* that even a well-funded, well-run, small hospital like Chestnut Lodge could exacerbate mental illness. He even had a theory how this happened, as explained in a chapter titled "Pathological Excitement and Hidden Staff Disagreement." "Whenever a patient showed manic excitement, he was always the subject of disagreement between two people who were often unaware of their own disagreement," the authors wrote. Stanton showed that tiny misunderstandings between bit players on the ward—a nurse forgetting to tell a patient where her clothes had been hung up was one of his famous examples—could cause great turmoil among incarcerated schizophrenics. Small events could prompt patients to "tear the ward apart," the authors noted, adding, "If the ward is put back together, the manic state will disappear."

Alfred Stanton's assignment was to drag McLean, kicking and screaming if necessary, into the twentieth century.

∽

What confronted Stanton and his team of Young Turks was "Dickensian," according to Dr. Merton Kahne, one of the doctors who followed Stanton into his new job. Horses and cows, left over from the days of the fully operational farm, still roamed the grounds. Some nurses and aides chose not to accept Social Security payments, so certain were they that McLean would always provide for them. "A great deal of nursing time was spent in taking care of things like sending gifts to people, sending flowers, writing thank-you notes, getting the fur coats off to storage when the summer came around," Kahne recalls. "The nurses had to make sure they didn't lose a coat—that was a very important thing." When he expressed interest in seeing an occupational therapy class, he was led into a small, airless room behind the hospital auditorium. "There were these old ladies rolling cloth into tampons. God knows how long that had been going on." Almost half the patient population was over seventy-five; the hospital had become a dumping ground for wealthy families to warehouse gaga Uncle Milton.

Things changed, and quickly. In a symbolic gesture, Stanton chose to live in Wellesley rather than to move his family into the baronial superintendent's residence. Stanton immediately hired a full-time psychologist—a woman no less—charged with building a professional department to backstop the medically trained analysts. He also brought on board a chief of social work, who in turn hired a raft of social workers to help manage the complex relations between the hospital and patients' families. And Stanton beefed up the residency training program, with the intention of luring top-quality medical students out to the sleepy Belmont campus.

A number of small changes in patients' lives had a cumulative impact. The disturbed wards had high fences surrounding modest yards; the new regime took them down. Stanton extended visiting time from a few hours a day to all daylight hours. For the first time, male nurses worked on female wards and vice versa. Patients finally gained access to telephones and no longer had to sign a pledge of good conduct to receive off-grounds "privileges"—a term Stanton loathed. The new doctors even allowed pets onto the halls, a reform eventually rescinded in the face of strenuous objections from the nurses, who had to clean up after the animals.

But most importantly, Stanton and his crew changed the way McLean cared for its patients. He did not believe in electroshock therapy or insulin shock therapy, and he never approved a lobotomy. Stanton did not believe in doping patients into a zombie-like state because it rendered them insensitive to the one cure he truly believed in: Freudian-style talk therapy. "He thought if you were really a good psychiatrist, you'd try to cure without drugs," remembers Washburn, one of Stanton's first trainees. "But if things got bad enough,"–Washburn laughs at the memory–"you could use drugs."* Never mind that Freud himself thought most schizophrenics dwelled well beyond the reach of psychoanalysis; Stanton thought otherwise. He committed his ideas to paper in an *Atlantic Monthly* article published in 1961, "Schizophrenics Can Recover." The article, which had been stage-managed by Stanton and the McLean trustees to commemorate the hospital's 150th anniversary, never really specified just how schizophrenics could "recover," but it assigned Stanton a great deal of credit for thinking that they could. It even quoted an unintentionally comic exchange between Stanton and his mentor, Sullivan:

> "Damn it Harry," [Stanton] said to Dr. Sullivan. "Schizophrenia is not all that tough. It should be easy to cure. We have been missing the point."
>
> Sullivan was attentive. "What makes you say that?"
>
> Stanton suddenly felt helpless. He could not remember the point.

The point was that there was no point. Neither Alfred Stanton in 1961 nor his successors in the twenty-first century had or has a workable program to "cure" schizophrenics or help them "recover." But Stanton was more than eager to try.

The new approach began the moment patients walked, or were wheeled, in the door. Previously, admission to McLean involved filling out a series of index cards. Stanton instituted the modern

---

*Yet McLean contributed significantly to the psychiatric drug revolution. In 1953, McLean's Dr. Willis Bower published the results of the first U.S. clinical trial of Thorazine, an antipsychotic drug that had gained widespread acceptance in Europe. Partly on the strength of Bower's enthusiastic write-up in the *New England Journal of Medicine*, Thorazine–hailed as a "chemical lobotomy" or "chemical straitjacket"–became the drug of choice in mental hospitals across America.

"work-up," which sometimes consumed three weeks and culminated in a thirty-page report. In seemingly endless interviews, young residents ran patients' life stories through complex theoretical "grids," looking for clues about the origins of his or her illness. "Stanton felt that if you did a really lengthy history, you'd understand the problem," says Washburn. "The idea was that you could see a life pattern, and the psychodynamic diagnosis would hit you in the face." The work-ups, integral to McLean's minimum-stay forty-day commitment policy, were hell on the residents and hell on some patients as well. When she checked herself into McLean in the mid-1960s, "I wanted to start working on my problems and start getting over them," Alice Brock remembers. "But no, the first few months, they've got to observe you, and test you, and observe you, and test you, and *then* they decide on some kind of treatment, and *then* they assign you a therapist, and *then* you actually go into therapy."

Every new case was discussed every day, for several weeks running, at staff conferences run by either Stanton or Kahne, a strict taskmaster who quickly became known as "Genghis" Kahne. "All the residents used to shake in fear of him," recalls Dr. Peter Choras. "He would say, 'Tell me a problem,' but it had to be a problem that was tough. So we'd present a tough problem, and he would say, 'I want every one of you guys to give me a different way of managing this.' When you got around the table to the fifth or sixth person, how many new ideas could you come up with to solve the same problem? It was scary."*

Stanton abhorred the laissez-faire McLean culture that allowed patients to publicly indulge their bizarre eccentricities without any intervention from the staff. These were the notorious "mu-

---

*Kahne's title of director of residency training carried other duties as well. There is a 1961 memo in the McLean files over his signature, laying down the ground rules for use of the tennis courts and golf course by the young trainees. Tennis was available to the resident doctors only in the morning before 9 A.M. "The golf course may be used at any time during the day or evening," Kahne wrote. "Because the course is small and pedestrians walk through the playing area, golfers are requested to adhere to safety rules, and heed the warning call of 'Fore.'"

seum pieces of pathology," some of whom did try to roam the grounds nude. One woman had what we would now call a shopping disorder. She filled her suite with boxes of clothes ordered from Jordan's and R.H. Stearns. When McLean staffers phoned her family to send some of the boxes home, they refused to take any; the lady in question had been sending merchandise to them as well. Another elderly dowager was allowed to roam the grounds dressed in the flowing blue gowns of a Thomas Gainsborough portrait. According to Washburn, "Stanton called in the young residents, and said, 'You are going along with psychopathology to allow this lady in blue to make a farce of herself. This is nothing to laugh about.' And suddenly going along with craziness began to go out of fashion."

The aim was to mobilize every patient, even the raving lunatics. One Stanton disciple conducted hour-long therapy sessions while her patients were immobilized in packs: shrouds of cold, wet sheets wrapped around the entire body. "Stanton analyzed the most psychotic patient I'd ever seen," remembers Choras. "He had her on the couch five days a week! That was rubbish—complete rubbish."

∞

In the summer of 1997, *I traveled to Nantucket to speak with Ruth* Tiffany Barnhouse, who did her psychiatric residency at McLean from 1953 to 1955, just as Alfred Stanton moved to Belmont. By the time I visited her, Barnhouse was a flinty, elegant lady in her eighties who smoked Nat Sherman cigarettes—and drew hostile stares—while we talked on a bench outside of Arno's, a bustling fern bar on the island's main drag. Barnhouse, who had left psychiatry to enter the Episcopal ministry and eventually taught at divinity school, was a strong believer in the mysteries of healing. Once inside the restaurant, I ordered the "Healthy Beginnings" brunch, and Dr. Barnhouse sneered. "I just refuse on principle to order any food that has the word 'health' in its description. The world began to go to hell in a basket when they substituted margarine for butter." When we started talking about the hospital administration of the 1950s, Barnhouse could not remember the name of her former boss. "He was a big name and a jerk," she said.

> He didn't want to put anybody on those psychotropic drugs—that was low—he preferred to just talk to people. He was a psychoanalytic nut. I had one girl, a very, very sick girl who was alcoholic, suicidal, and a lesbian with a multiple personality disorder. She was terribly sick and in and out of the hospital. She was quite intelligent, and this guy would say, "Well, when she's through treatment, she'll go to college and this and this," and that was just dumb. He could say that stuff and mean it, it was really weird. He hired a bunch of analysts and hired social workers and all that stuff.

Of course, she meant Alfred Stanton.

"Alfred Stanton." Barnhouse's friend and former colleague Robert Coles lingered on the name when I interviewed him in a noisy coffee shop not far from his house in Concord, Massachusetts. Coles, now a well-known writer and child psychologist, was a young psychiatric resident at McLean when Stanton came on the scene. "He represented so-called progress," Coles recalled. "He brought in all the baggage of the wretched mid-twentieth century and totally messed up McLean. That was the beginning of the end":

> When I came to the hospital in the mid-fifties, Stanton had just taken over. I was a young man, but I immediately identified with the old order, which is a little unusual. For some reason I didn't like what they were doing, which was taking over this hospital whose ways and manners I liked. The residents there hadn't really been regarded as psychiatric patients in the full twentieth-century sense of that phrase, which

I felt had a reductionist and patronizing connotation at the hands of some of these talkers.

George Eliot uses this term in *Middlemarch:* "the Christian carnivore." These were the shrink carnivores. They were examining every nook and crevice, they were just devastating that hospital. Maybe some of that had some salutary effects, but I thought it was hurting a lot of people. I mean, there used to be a nice golf course, there were nice tennis courts, and suddenly all this was taking second fiddle to group meetings. . . . Here you have patients who have grown up in a world of stoic silence and privacy, and suddenly you have doctors who are coming "at" you and want to get you to talk and talk and talk. And then you find out they're talking about you in the library, which no longer is a library most of the day, because they're having meetings here starting at eight o'clock in the morning.

You couldn't do anything without having an hour or two of "thought." There was pervasive self-consciousness that expressed itself in the most portentous, dreary language that I just thought was a lot of smog and fog. I identified with some of the patients there, whose idiosyncrasies and ways of dressing and talking I kind of liked. We drank tea, ate food, we chatted. I remember having a discussion about "General Eisenhower" with a man who said, "I don't like to call him president, he's president because he's a general." Then he went into this long discussion that I thought was very well argued. I was impressed with this mobilization of intellect by a man you could dismiss as a manic depressive, which is what he was in the prelithium era.

The patients were not without resources when commenting on what Coles, in an allusion to Hitler's Germany, calls Stanton's "New Order." In 1958, the Patient Activities Association staged an elaborate musical, written by two patients, called *Close to Home.*

Scored to original music, *Close to Home* is an hour-long parody of life at the Belmont Hill Bettering House, where patients just want to be loved, but doctors insist on analyzing them. The protagonist, Andy, has a drinking problem that has landed him a stay at the Bettering House. After belting out his opening number, "The Forty-Day Commitment Blues," Andy meets the pair of young psychiatric residents assigned to his case, who have been practicing inscrutable stares in front of a mirror before his arrival.

BOTH: *We are brimming full of questions*
                       In our aggravating way
                       With an enervating come-back
                       To anything you say . . .
                       We gesticulate with glasses
                       Primly puff upon our pipes
                       As we make our diagnosis
                       Casting you into type.

The shrinks quickly segue into their "Diagnostic Tango":

BOTH: *It began by suppression*
                       Went on to repression
                       Causing regression
                       To covert aggression
                       And overt depression
                       There's quite clearly displacement
                       With ego replacement
                       Simple denial
                       That Life is a trial
                       And all remaining is id.

2ND PSYCH.:   *Yes!*

BOTH: *And all remaining is id.*

1ST PSYCH.:   *There is symptom conversion*
                       A dash of perversion

> *Some introjection*
> *And ample projection*
> *Back to the womb he has slid.*

2ND PSYCH.: *Yes!*

BOTH: *Back to the womb he has slid.*

1ST PSYCH.: *There is thought dereistic*
And daydreams autistic
Oddball delusion
That life is illusion
He's slightly loose in the lid.

2ND PSYCH.: *Yes!*

BOTH: *He's slightly loose in the lid. OLE!*

Psychiatrist Number 2 clearly got good grades at Harvard Medical School. He is awarded a solo in which he explains that all thinking can be reduced to mere "mental mechanisms":

> *In this age of automation*
> *Thought is free association*
> *Anna Freud's hallucination*
> *Tells us how our minds are made. . . .*
> *A change of heart, reaction formation*
> *Admiration is idealization*
> *When love's no more than identification*
> *This formulation or symbolization*
> *Is one big hell of a rationalization.*
> *Dreams are just dissociation*
> *Memories—incorporation*
> *Fear, of course, invokes castration*
> *Or vice versa may be said.*

The patient characters are a genial collection of McLean oddballs. Andy's new friend Homer has been in the hospital forever. "I wouldn't think of leaving," he says.

HOMER: I love it here. It's great. Tennis. Occupational therapy. Evening entertainments of universally outstanding quality.

ANDY: How come they don't just sort of kick you out?

HOMER: I can generally tell when they are about to suggest it again. Then I just think up something rather horrifying for my therapist. You know, something rare. A nice traumatic primal scene. It works every time.

Addie, one of the two female leads, is the "Belle of Belmont Hill." She confesses to "primitive instincts":

> *Beautiful Belle of Belmont Hill*
> *Truly unruly morally*
> *Sex is the vexing core of me*
> *Seeking a Jack to be his Jill. . . .*
> *Horribly boring being coy*
> *Shyly beguiling smiles are bunk*
> *Better if sweater and shorts have shrunk*
> *My standard ploy: "I WANT A BOY!"*

Close to Home ends happily. The shiftless Homer works up the courage to leave the Bettering House and takes Addie with him. Andy and his girlfriend Cassie sing a beautiful duet, "In Love, Sort Of," and decide to ask the psychiatrists if they can leave Belmont to start a new life together. In the face of so much true love, even the shrinks briefly shed their forbidding masks, singing that "everyone is human after all." They graciously release Cassie and Andy, who reprise their love duet with these lines:

> *Hello, farewell,*
> *Nothing seems to last*

Live now, love now
Before the dream has passed.
Can we tell what comes tomorrow
No, no. Our time we must borrow
We are in love,
Truly, in love.

Close to Home was a great success, playing to packed houses on three separate evenings in the Pierce Hall auditorium. The show even went on the road, to the Austen Riggs sanitarium in Stockbridge, Massachusetts. There was talk of going to New York, if not to Broadway then perhaps to Bellevue or to the Bloomingdale Asylum. In real life, alas, not all endings are happy. The *Close to Home* story ends on a mixed note, combining the grievous and felicitous events that make up real life in a mental hospital. The female librettist committed suicide. Composer Sam Heilner, who played the piano during the show, later returned to his job at the *Boston Globe*.*

∽

Alfred Stanton had his critics; he had them all his life. But there is no doubt that he succeeded in introducing McLean to the twentieth century. Not only did he modernize patient care at the hospital, but he also laid the groundwork for future innovations. He helped launch the day care, or outpatient, program, an important change for a hospital that had always viewed itself as a high-class

---

*The *Globe* published a lengthy obituary when its revered, longtime employee passed away in 1982, and although it did mention his "psychiatric afflictions," it did not record his coauthorship of *Close to Home*. Choate- and Harvard-educated, rich, a witty raconteur and a mixer of ferocious dry martinis, Heilner was a classic McLean consumer. His friend and colleague Jack Thomas recalls that Heilner, upon learning of a threatened strike at the newspaper, immediately checked himself into McLean. "He explained that he had a panic attack," Thomas says. "'I couldn't stand the idea of no structure,' was what he said."

hotel for the mentally afflicted. In the 1960s and 1970s, medical insurers would come to favor such partial-payment, nonresidential plans over the costlier inpatient schemes. Gradually, Stanton changed the demographics of the inpatient population, refusing to let his asylum become a storage facility for batty Brahmins and reaching out to different, more-challenging cases. As the 1960s progressed, he correctly deduced that troubled young people might benefit from sojourns at McLean and that affluent parents would be willing to finance them. It was on Stanton's watch that McLean opened the Arlington School, an accredited high school for boys and girls living inside and outside the hospital. Just as important, he traveled the country, jawboning government and private funding agencies for grants and promoting McLean as a first-class teaching hospital of national renown.

But his tenure at the helm of McLean ended on a plaintive note, following two successive, apparently uncontrollable waves of suicides. Although the deaths were never mentioned in the hospital's annual reports, they were described as an "epidemic" in published research papers.

Psychiatrists who worked at McLean in the early 1960s have trouble remembering the precise dates of the suicides because they spiked in two different years. Six patients killed themselves during the 1961/1962 academic year, and then seven committed suicide in 1965/1966. In between the two spikes, there were seven additional suicides. These were very high numbers for a 250-patient hospital. Dr. George Lawson, a McLean psychiatrist, distributed an informal paper in 1966 that put McLean's numbers in context—a context that amounted to a scathing indictment of the Stanton regime. From 1936 until 1956, the year Stanton arrived, McLean experienced seven suicides, an average rate of 0.35 a year. In the first decade of Stanton's regime, Lawson wrote, "thirty-six people have died by suicide who were either patients of the hospital or intimately connected with its treatment programs." So suicides had increased tenfold under Stanton, and the rate compared unfavorably with that of other mental hospitals. "The present rate of 3.6 [suicides a year] is three times higher than the overall mental hospital average, or a rate of 150 times higher than the general population," according to Lawson. "Stanton had advertised to the psychiatric world that if you can't take care of the desperately ill, we can at McLean," recalls one doctor. "So many patients arrived there having failed at Shepherd Pratt or at Chestnut Lodge. They arrived with the expectation that they had come to the best mental hospital in the world, and when they began to fail, they were hopeless."

Stanton himself, a cool customer in staff conferences and in one-on-one analyses, was distraught by the suicides and the impact they were having on his hospital's reputation. In response, he committed what many consider to have been a cardinal error: He tightened his supervision over the ward administrators. By so doing, he broadcast his concern about the deaths. But at the same time, he instructed his subordinates never to discuss the suicides with the patients, who were of course fully informed through the hospital grapevine. "Stanton behaved in the most uncharacteristic way of not wanting to discuss it," says Irene Stiver, the woman whom Stanton hired as the hospital's first clinical psychologist. "He was afraid that the situation would escalate if you allowed people to talk about it. I think it was very poor clinical judgment, but he was the psychiatrist-in-chief and he was the one responsible. He got into this crazy thing about how we couldn't even bring the subject up at conferences."

Some psychiatrists lied to their patients about the suicides, and some did not. The patients picked up on this conflict immediately; indeed, it is precisely the kind of destabilizing disagreement described in Stanton's book *The Mental Hospital.* "The preoccupation with the avoidance of suicide is so great that it is immediately and accurately telegraphed to the patients, which places a dreadful weapon in the service of their anger," Lawson wrote in his critique. And the more disturbed patients were perfectly willing to wield the weapon. Even patients who were monitored twelve times an hour on five-minute "checks" managed to kill themselves. Suicide pacts arose; two women swallowed cyanide in the kitchen of an apartment where their therapists allowed them to live. A group of young women on South Belknap, the ward that Susanna Kaysen would later make famous in her book *Girl, Interrupted,* branded themselves the "OSS girls": "Over-Sexed, Over Sixteen, and Over-Suicidal." A young man hanged himself inside Eliot Chapel. "They said he should have hung himself on the sign outside McLean," one administrator remembers, "because that's what the hospital specialized in."

Stanton assigned his trusted deputy Kahne to probe the causes of the suicides. Kahne ended up publishing four papers on the subject, which echoed some of the key lessons in *The Mental Hospital.* "The central theme that I got out of it was when the strength of the relational system was diminished, chances of suicide were very high," Kahne told me years later. "For example, people were killing themselves in the middle of summer, when the academic residents were leaving and there was tremendous personnel turnover."

Kahne concluded that the rapid pace of change at McLean was destabilizing patients' lives. Even with the average length of stay plummeting to less than four months, 40 percent of the patients were having their cases shuffled among different social workers during their stay. Many of the older doctors were cutting back their hours at the hospital, increasing the workload on the young residents drafted into the hospital. Stanton had eliminated the traditional admissions unit, for instance, placing new patients directly into wards. Stanton wanted to spare patients the disruption of a move during their stay, but often the new arrivals, experiencing a mental hospital for the first time, roiled ward life.

In another change, new, inexperienced nurses were assigned to the disturbed wards instead of being allowed a breaking-in period in a more tranquil setting. And the new McLean was growing very big. In just a few years, Stanton had increased McLean's professional staff—doctors, psychologists, and social workers—tenfold, from ten to one hundred. "People would be killing themselves when the aides and the personnel didn't even know their names, because they hadn't had time to learn them," Kahne said. "I suggested that they slow down the turnover or try out different hiring procedures."

Kahne also interviewed the McLean psychiatrists who had lost patients to suicide—doctors whose patients had "fired" them, in the dark vernacular of the hospital wardroom. They criticized the administration's panicked reaction to each suicide: "All decisions seemed to have been reduced to one overriding concern—to insure the passage of about 72 hours without another death." Change itself, it seemed, was killing them:

> As the "epidemic" of suicides wore on, the most prominent ethos about the cause of the epidemic, which increasingly pervaded the opinions of most therapists (including those who had had a patient commit suicide) . . . was that there was an excessive moral demand for the patients to change their way of living and that this had become so much an implicit part of the social expectations that patients unable to meet the demand experienced intense guilt. The guilt was believed to be so intense for some as to cost their lives.

As it happens, Stanton had allowed a professional sociologist, Rose Coser, free access to McLean during the early 1960s so that she could write a book on the residency training of young psychiatrists. "While she was doing her interviews, there was also this incredible suicide epidemic going on," recalls Harold Williams, who started working at McLean in 1962. "So she had a front seat on that arena and could tap into everybody's ongoing feelings."

In the middle of the suicide wave, Coser chronicled a sense of cynicism and despair among the residents. From her interviews, she learned that Stanton continually postponed his scheduled weekly meetings with the first-year residents—unless there had been a suicide. One resident told her, "You'll be interested to know that Dr. X [Stanton] has canceled again. This is the fourth time. What we need is another suicide. (Smiles uncomfortably.)"

Coser then asked Stanton if she could examine his appointment calendar. Initially taken aback, he opened up his appointment books for the six years of her study. She correlated his frequent absences, and the sense of abandonment among the residents, with suicides at the hospital.

"Whenever Stanton went away, he got really nervous, because he was leaving his post and we wild guys were going to be running the hospital," Williams recalled. "That's when he would say, 'You guys are playing Russian roulette with five chambers loaded,' stuff like that, which made you feel really good. The more he said that, the more he drove down confidence and self-esteem, and the more our knuckles got white on the joystick." Tense and overreactive when in his office and a poor delegator outside the office, Alfred Stanton was running a dysfunctional hospital.

McLean was almost twice as large as Chestnut Lodge, where Stanton and Schwartz had conducted their groundbreaking research. The suicides, some of them children of prominent families, were prompting difficult inquiries from the hospital's trustees. Furthermore, McLean was running a deficit, which had to be funded by other Harvard teaching hospitals. Under pressure, Stanton appointed a director of hospital affairs and then created and filled the new position of clinical director to insulate himself from the running of the hospital. As any reader of *The Mental Hospital* might have predicted, the agitation did not help matters any. The abrupt resignation of the freshly minted clinical director, who correctly perceived that he had been brought on as a flak-catcher, triggered what may have been a mental institution first: a full-dress, placard-waving ("Bring Back Sam Silverman!") patient demonstration in front of the administration building. In the following academic year, 1965/1966, seven more suicides occurred at McLean.

Pressured from many sides, Stanton gave up running the hospital and concentrated instead on psychiatric research. In an act of almost gratuitous cruelty, Harvard denied him a coveted endowed professorship that Stanton thought he had been promised. "He had the energy of Niagara Falls, but later his enthusiasm faded," says Peter Choras. "Alfred never lived up to his promise, although his brilliance was always there." Dr. Edward Daniels points to McLean's impossible parking situation as evidence of Stanton's signal achievement: getting McLean going again. "When he came, there used to be six cars parked in front of the administration building. Now all the lots are full." But like most of his colleagues, Daniels gives Stanton mixed reviews: "Stanton had a way of being preoccupied with tiny details. . . . he could immerse himself for a week in a nonsensical hunk of nothing." In the middle of the first suicide wave, Stanton issued this memo, to which he twice affixed his psychiatrist-in-chief stamp:

OFFICIAL NOTICE; File Under: H
TO: All Physicians and Nursing Personnel
SUBJECT: Hot Water Bottles

Effective at once, the use of hot water bottles as medical procedure is to be discontinued at McLean Hospital.

December 13, 1961

In questions of administration, Stanton could simply get lost. Longtime facilities manager Henry Langevin remembers presenting Stanton with three competing bids for resurfacing McLean's central tennis court, where Stanton himself often played. But the director was paralyzed by indecision because the switch from the clay to a hard surface would eliminate a cherished job—rolling and sweeping the ochre-colored clay—for one of the hospital's elderly, chronic schizophrenics. "What's poor Elmer going to do?" was Stanton's plaint, as the trivial court resurfacing decision hung fire for months. Yet "when he gave a conference on a major problem patient, it could have been recorded and published, it was so good," according to Daniels. "His failure was not in his clinical work; his failure was in the very thing he specialized in, in interpersonal relationships."

It was a terrible paradox: The man who wrote the book on mental hospitals proved to be not terribly adroit at running one.

∽

Alfred Stanton's career was to have one more interesting twist. He surrendered the title of psychiatrist-in-chief in 1967 and devoted the next fifteen years to research. During that time, he raised money, recruited doctors, and oversaw one of the most ambitious psychiatric research projects ever undertaken, a project that would scuttle one of his own most cherished beliefs: that intensive psychotherapy could help deeply disturbed, schizophrenic patients.

When *Effects of Psychotherapy in Schizophrenia, I and II* was finally published in 1984, the book-length work claimed nine authors, and the research had engaged eighty-one therapists and 164 patients from five major teaching hospitals, including McLean. Stanton played the role of honcho-godfather-coordinator for the study, which took over a decade to design and implement. He left the heavy lifting to Dr. John Gunderson, an ambitious and intelligent young psychoanalyst just beginning a research career in the field of borderline personality disorders. The timing of the schizophrenia study was crucial. The psychopharmaceutical revolution had just begun. For the first time, doctors realized that comparatively cheap drug regimens might hold out more promise for treating, or at least stabilizing, disturbed patients than psychoanalysis. "This was at the beginning of the rift within psychiatry between the psychodynamic and the biological people," Gunderson explained to me in his office at Bowditch Hall. "Before we started there had already been three studies that failed to show much benefit from psychotherapy, but they were flawed. What was needed was a really definitive study—enter us."

Although the logistics of quantifying the purported progress of an unstable sample of 164 schizophrenic patients were daunting—sixty-nine subjects dropped out within six months—the research design was relatively simple. Two groups of schizophrenic patients would be assigned different kinds of therapy: One was the Sullivan/Fromm-Reichmann type of intensive psychotherapy, called EIO, or exploratory, insight-oriented therapy, administered three times a week. The other patients received a more modern treatment called RAS, or reality-adaptive supportive psychotherapy, offered once a week or less. The aim of the insight therapy, the study explained, was "to explore the patient's inner life," often using the traditional Freudian tools such as discussions of family history, childhood traumas, and so on. RAS was something else. It was deemed to be more "present-oriented" and more practical, "intended to identify problems that could be solved or that could be expected to recur in the future. . . . Another major feature of the RAS therapy was its focus on the patient's behavior itself rather than the potential covert meanings behind the behavior." Perhaps most importantly, it "provided patients with a coherent theory about their illness which emphasized its biological origins and the need for long-term, largely pharmacologic treatment."

The authors buried their conclusions beneath the usual mound of academic qualifiers, for example: "There is no easy way to reduce the results into a single statement that one form of therapy is preferential to another." But the message came through loud and clear. "Obviously the results failed to confirm either the strength or breadth of favorable effects that we hypothesized would be associated with the EIO as opposed to the RAS treatment," they wrote. Translation: Occasional, supportive sessions with carefully medicated schizophrenics yielded the same results as expensive, staff-intensive psychotherapy. "Equally important was the finding that by some external standard, most notably time spent outside of a hospital and in full-time employment, the RAS therapy emerged as the preferable form of treatment." This, the authors conceded, was "clearly the single most convincing finding of the study." Translation: Modern psychiatric management could get schizophrenics not only out of the hospital but even into jobs! No, the patients probably wouldn't return to their labs at MIT or to the Harvard lecture hall, but they might be able to work in an academic library or hold down a job as a research assistant in a white-collar office.

The study had a huge impact on psychiatry. "I don't think our study showed that psychotherapy can't be effective, or is never effective," Gunderson says. "A safer interpretation is that it can't be counted on to be effective. But in the larger psychiatric community, the message was that insight-oriented psychotherapy won't help schizophrenic patients. So that approach wilted on the vine overnight—within a few years it was not practiced or taught in medical school." Its impact on Stanton was less clear. He died one year before the study was published, although of course he was familiar with the results. At weekly meetings with Gunderson, he would analyze, reanalyze, and overanalyze their research findings, prevaricating madly in the same way that he managed to stave off the decision about resurfacing the tennis court. "He would always wrap up these meetings by saying, 'We've decided that a decision is not possible,'" Gunderson recalls. "It drove me absolutely crazy. He was a mild, sweet man who liked intellectual discourse, but he lacked productivity. He liked research, but he didn't really want answers."

∞

Alfred Stanton is almost completely unknown to the world of modern psychiatry. The Mental Hospital is no longer required reading in medical schools. Patients today rarely stay on wards long enough to develop the kind of covert conflicts that Stanton and Schwartz took such pains to document in 1954. At McLean, Stanton's career went into rapid eclipse in the mid-1960s when the hospital began running up deficits, attributed mainly to his lack of administrative ability. Ever since Gilbert Stuart painted John McLean, the hospital has commissioned portraits of its directors and top benefactors and awarded them pride of place in the administration building.

Stanton's portrait was relegated to the Alfred Stanton Room in Higginson House, where many of McLean's "attending," or part-time, doctors had their offices. After a few years, the elegant sitting room was carved up into secretarial cubicles, and Stanton's portrait was removed to the hospital library. The land under Higginson House has been sold, and it will soon be torn down to make way for an office park.

Ironically—because Gunderson confesses to having mixed feelings about Stanton—he is the executor of a small endowment that organizes an annual dinner and lecture in Stanton's memory. In the present era of all psychopharmaceutical all the time, Gunderson remains firmly committed to psychosocial therapy, or talk therapy, as a primary mode of healing. A full professor in the Harvard system, he is also McLean's director of psychosocial research services.

Gunderson invited me to attend the Stanton Lecture, which was preceded by a dinner at the Harvard Faculty Club. Of the twenty-five attendees, only a handful had actually known Stanton. The rest were therapists in their late forties and early fifties who may have stood in the back of the room during a Stanton patient "consult" or who perhaps remembered his name from medical school. The lecturer, Daniel Stern, an American expert on mother-child development with an appointment in Geneva, admitted that he had never heard of Alfred Stanton until his invitation arrived in the mail. When Stern spoke at McLean the following day, Gunderson joked to the overflow audience in Pierce Hall that "the Alfred Stanton Lectures have become better known than Alfred Stanton himself."

The dinner resembled a meeting of the Last of the Mohicans. As always, the Harvard Faculty Club atmosphere was subdued and elegant in the downbeat, academic manner; the wine was drinkable and the sautéed chicken breast in basil sauce a full cut above rubbery institutional fare. The bar was open, but in public company, psychiatrists drink carefully. As the evening wore on, the men and women toasted the threatened ideal of "talk therapy." The talk even turned to Freud's famous (to this audience) analysis of the paranoid Judge Schreiber, a genuine museum piece of psychiatric history. One therapist noted sardonically that he practices in "the last bastion of long-term care": a prison hospital for the criminally insane. The old-timers glumly swapped medical updates. Irene Stiver, whom Stanton chose as McLean's first clinical psychologist, had passed away. Harold Williams had suffered a stroke. No one was precisely sure if Harriet Stanton, Alfred's widow, was living in Virginia or had moved to a rest home in Florida. I had spoken to Stanton's two surviving children during the past year and shared my information.

A little wine brought forth the customary reminiscences. Golda Edinburg, McLean's retired chief of social work, remembered that the straitlaced Stanton had taken her and several colleagues to a striptease show in San Francisco during a business trip, all in the service of broadening horizons. A psychiatrist recalled a crowded patient consultation from the mid-1970s, when a perplexing case was presented to a group of McLean doctors, with Stanton in attendance. The presenting physician was describing his patient's sexual fantasies and seeking therapeutic guidance. In some detail, the doctor told how this man wanted to get down on all fours and crawl around the streets of Boston, sniffing the rear ends of all the attractive women he met. The presentation was greeted with silence; even a full decade into the so-called sexual revolution, a certain squeamishness prevailed when bow-tied Harvard doctors assembled in a room. After a few moments, it was Stanton's voice that broke the silence: "And did the patient think this behavior was *normal?*" he asked. The tension dissolved; Stanton laughed; the doctors laughed. Psychiatry continued on its appointed rounds.

8

The Mad Poets' Society

> . . . I feel like a periwinkle
> Left too high on the beach
> By the tide . . .
> What flood was it
> That brought me here?
>
> **Eleanor Morris, "Easter Sunday"**

The poet Anne Sexton thought that writing poetry kept her sane.
Shortly after her first suicide attempt at age twenty-eight, Sexton was institutionalized at Westwood Lodge, a comfortable sanitarium not far from her home in Wellesley, Massachusetts. While recuperating, Sexton met a talented young musician who was also a patient of her psychiatrist, Dr. Martin Orne. "I was thrilled to get into the Nut House," Sexton later told a friend. "I found this girl (very crazy of course) (like me I guess) who talked language." By "language," Sexton meant the bold, figurative language of poetry. According to Sexton's biographer Diane Middlebrook, the

poet created her own Genesis myth, as a writer "born again" from the trough of despair. "I found I belonged to the poets," Sexton said, and with the encouragement of her psychiatrist, she started writing poetry. Dr. Orne responded generously to her first baby steps into her incipient profession. "He said they were wonderful," Sexton recalled. "I kept writing and writing and giving them all to him. . . . I kept writing because he was approving." Middlebrook concludes: "Poetry had saved her life."

Sexton had another idée fixe: She wanted to be admitted to McLean. "I want a scholarship to McLean," Sexton confided to her longtime friend and amanuensis Lois Ames, as if she was talking about a fellowship to the American Academy of Arts and Science. Sexton certainly had the qualifications: Two suicide attempts by the age of thirty; extended stays at the Glenside and Westwood Lodge sanitariums. She wrote about her mania in her first poetry collection, *To Bedlam and Part Way Back.* She reveled, theatrically, in her madness and was not above exploiting her shocking mood swings to manipulate her friends and family. But Dr. Orne, wary of McLean's high prices and extended stays, refused to commit her there. Sexton had won the Pulitzer Prize and been profiled in national magazines. But she had never punched her ticket at McLean.

Why McLean? Because of Sylvia Plath and Robert Lowell. "We both recognized that Plath and Lowell had been there, and she wanted to be in that lineage," Ames says. "The same way she wanted to be buried in Mt. Auburn cemetery, where her family was buried." Sexton was ferociously competitive with Plath in all respects. Both had been reared in Boston's well-to-do western suburbs. Both women were fearfully articulate, beautiful, and sexually alert. They had both committed themselves to big poetry, publishing in the big magazines (*The New Yorker, Atlantic Monthly*) and with the big publishing houses (Knopf and Houghton Mifflin), and to winning the big awards (the Yale Younger Poets Award, the Pulitzer Prize). Each knew she was unstable and vaguely understood that psychological torment somehow produced good poetry. Both saw themselves—correctly—as future suicides. Meeting in drunken martini klatches at the Ritz Hotel following Lowell's Boston University poetry seminar, the two femmes fatales even discussed killing themselves. (Sexton on Plath: "She told the story of her first suicide in sweet and loving detail.") The conversation was never hypothetical. When talking about suicide, Plath and Sexton were not interested in questions of "if" or "when" but of "how." After Plath died, Sexton published a bitchy essay/poem, griping that Plath had trumped her in their mortal combat:

> *Thief!*
> *how did you . . . crawl down alone*
> *into the death I wanted so badly and for so long.*

The experiences of Lowell, a mentor of sorts, weighed heavily in Sexton's thinking too. Although deeply versed in classical poetry, Lowell wrote in a beautiful American vernacular, and he wrote about life as he found it, whether it be an uncompromising portrait of his ineffectual father ("Father's death was abrupt and unprotesting") or a heartrending description of returning to his wife and daughter after a few months in the "bin" ("I keep no rank nor station / Cured, I am frizzled, stale and small"). As a student in his class, she could not help but notice that he disappeared around Christmas time, sometimes to McLean, when his mania overwhelmed him. One of Sexton's first recognized poems describes the ungainly Lowell, "like a hunk of big frog," leaving his crowded poetry seminar to make the trip to the hospital grounds in suburban Belmont: "I must admire your skill," Sexton wrote. "You are so gracefully insane."

By the time he first checked in to McLean in 1958, Robert Lowell was, as they say in the consumer-products field, a repeat user. Forty-one years old, a Pulitzer Prize winner, and one of the country's most respected poets, Lowell experienced uncontrollable manic surges and had been institutionalized before. To the astonishment of those around him, he would swell up with power, anger, and delusion. He would shower his closest friends with bitter, mocking curses or proclaim undying love to an airline stewardess and insist on leaving the plane with her to start a new life. He was capable of delivering a gibbering lecture lauding Adolf Hitler. Some stereotypes are true; there are people in mental institutions who want to assume the power of Napoleon or Jesus Christ, and at times Robert Lowell was one of them.

Robert Lowell was the uncrowned poet laureate of McLean just on the strength of his magnificent poem "Waking in the Blue"—excerpted at the front of this book.

"Waking" was included in the book *Life Studies,* which many Lowell scholars believe to be his best book. It is intensely autobiographical and unsparing of his immediate and extended family. One of the poet's cousins, Sarah Payne Stuart, has recently suggested that the family's hostility to the poems may have precipitated a breakdown that landed Lowell back at McLean. After reading a prepublication copy of the book, Lowell's formidable aunt Sarah Cotting announced that "I've just read what Bobby wrote about [his parents] Charlotte and Bob, and it's just awful." From her Beacon Hill town house, she marched downhill to Lowell's home on nearby Marlborough Street and gave her nephew a piece of her mind. (This was the same aunt who once mused, while sitting on her yacht: "Why doesn't Bobby write about the sea? It's so pretty.") "I'm sorry you didn't like it," Lowell answered softly. "I thought it was rather good." A few weeks later, when *Life Studies* was formally published, Lowell was at McLean.

Because he was born into the Boston aristocracy, Lowell understood instinctively who was in McLean and why. He had grown up with the "Mayflower screwballs"; the "thoroughbred mental cases"; "these victorious figures of bravado ossified young." No nuance of Boston snobbery could escape him, not least that he hailed from the line of thin-blooded—that is, creative—Lowells as opposed to the broad-shouldered, industrial-titan Lowells who enriched themselves from the textile mills along the Charles and Merrimack Rivers. Ralph Lowell, the downtown banker chairman of McLean's trustees, was a "real" Lowell. Robert and his family, although they lived quite comfortably, were comparatively poor relations. Robert's father, Robert Traill Spence Lowell III, was a middle-ranking naval officer who had made a good match. His wife's family, the Winslows, proudly traced their ancestry back to the Mayflower. The venerable names attached to the McLean halls—Wyman, Appleton, Higginson, and Bowditch—were the names of family friends. Robert had attended St. Mark's School with them, and they had gone on to Harvard too. Writing to his friend the poet Elizabeth Bishop, Lowell read the hospital like an open book, in this case the book being a crazy salad of a Marquand novel, the Harvard faculty directory, and the Social Register:

I live in an interesting house now at McLean's, one in which no man had entered since perhaps 1860; suddenly it was made co-ed. It was like entering some ancient deceased sultan's seraglio. We were treated to a maze of tender fussy attentions suitable for very old ladies: chocolate scented milk at 8:30; a lounging and snoozing bed read after meals, each announcement of an appointment gently repeated at ten minute intervals, an old crone waiting on table barking like television turned on full to pierce through deafness. On the other hand, it took three days to get a shaving glass.

The man next to me is a Harvard Law professor. One day, he is all happiness, giving the plots of Trollope novels, distinguishing delicately between the philosophies of Holmes and Brandeis, reminiscing wittily about Frankfurter. But on another day, his depression blankets him. Early in the morning, I hear cooing pigeon sounds, and if I listen carefully, the words: "Oh terror. TERROR!" Our other male assembles microscopically exact models of clippers and three masted schooners.

Both men, and I too, shrink before a garrulous Mrs. Churchill, sometimes related to the statesman and sometimes to the novelist. "How are you related to Thomas Arnold Lowell?" I assumed she meant James Russell Lowell, and was abysmally wrong and have never been to explain. Pointing to a classical moulding on a mantelpiece, she will say, "That's Cameron Forbes, the ambassador to Japan," or begin a dinner conversation with, "Speaking of Rhode Island reds . . . "

Sometimes with a big paper napkin stuck like an escaping bra on her throat, she will dance a little jig and talk about being presented to Queen Victoria. She was.

Lowell visited McLean four times over the course of eight years. Like Plath, he left a paper trail of letters with the distinctive return address "175 Mill Street, Belmont, Massachusetts." He is possibly the only patient to have exchanged letters from the wards with Jacqueline Kennedy; she thanked him for a book he had sent her and congratulated him on getting away for the holidays. Lowell also corresponded with the poet Theodore Roethke, who had his own struggles with mental illness (Lowell: "I feel great kinship with you"), and mailed a letter from Bowditch to Ezra Pound, who had been locked up in St. Elizabeth's Hospital in Washington, D.C. "Do you think a man who has been off his rocker as often as I have could run for elective office and win?" Lowell inquired of Pound.

I have in mind the state senatorship from my district—the South End, Back Bay Boston, and your son's Roxbury etc. The incumbent is an inconspicuous Republican. His rival is a standard losing party democrat. I'd run as a democrat, and if I could edge out in the very difficult primaries, then I'd cream the Republican. And then there'd be vistas before me as I sat in the Boston State Capitol on my little $5,000 a year job that would cost me about $10,000. What's your advice?

There is no trace of a reply.

Many of Lowell's students, some of whom became noted poets in their own right, trooped out to Belmont to visit their mentor. Some days, Lowell was very clear and his students would read to him from books he had requested, or they would share poetry, occasionally attracting a small crowd of not-very-aware patients. On other days, Lowell was in the mania, reworking famous poems in his copy of the *Norton Anthology* or retranslating, for naught, works from Greek and Latin. The students were suffused with sadness, seeing their brilliant teacher temporarily defeated by mental illness.

Poet Frank Bidart, a former student who became Lowell's friend and literary executor, recalls one visit:

> People knew he was a writer. He was an older person, and there were other older people there, as well as some kids in their twenties. There's a way in which the place and the circumstances became very egalitarian, each patient is just one more person with a roommate. There was no hierarchy. Lowell was fine with that. I think he was a little embarrassed at the beginning for me to see him like that, that he couldn't leave, that I had to bring him books. I mean, he could have worn shoes if he wanted to, but he didn't want to. He was living as if he were at the beach or something, but he wasn't at the beach.

Just before Alfred Stanton took over as psychiatrist-in-chief at McLean, Franklin Wood admitted a young woman who would become the hospital's first mass-market celebrity patient: an intelligent, troubled Smith College junior named Sylvia Plath. Writing about her suicide attempt in her novel *The Bell Jar*, Plath informed a generation of young women that one could suffer a nervous breakdown and live to write about it, in theory, at least.* Three weeks after its publication in Britain, in 1963, Plath killed herself. When it appeared in America eight years later, with its vivid descriptions of life on "Wymark" (Wyman) and "Belsize" (Belknap) halls, it became must reading for young girls, in the same way that J.D. Salinger's classic *Catcher in the Rye* was being devoured by moody, adolescent boys. In *The Bell Jar,* thousands of American teenagers were getting a firsthand look inside McLean, which, the twenty-one-year-old Plath told a friend, was "the best mental hospital in the U.S."

The story of Plath's stay at McLean has entered the literary canon not only by way of *The Bell Jar* but also from the pens of numerous biographers and memoirists. The consensus tale runs like this: Plath, a sensitive, erudite, and hard-working young woman from a conventional but not particularly happy family in Wellesley, Massachusetts, experienced mild depressions while studying at Smith College. As versed in Freud as any budding intellectual of her generation, she thought she had "penis envy" and suffered from "schizophrenia." After winning a prestigious national contest to work at *Mademoiselle* magazine in New York during July 1953, she suffered a rare career setback; she was denied admission to a Harvard summer writing seminar. Trapped at home in August, drained of energy, she began to contemplate suicide. After a half-serious attempt to drown herself during a beach picnic, Plath swallowed an overdose of her mother's sleeping pills and hid in a crawl space underneath her parents' home. She very nearly died. ("Beautiful Smith Girl Missing at Wellesley" and "Top Ranking Student at Smith Missing from Wellesley Home" were two of the front-page headlines in the Boston papers.) Her family and doctors properly concluded that her attempt exceeded the classic suicide gesture and packed her off to McLean.

---

*Four years after she checked out of McLean, Plath noted in her journal that a recent issue of *Cosmopolitan* magazine had two articles on mental health. "I *must* write one about a college girl suicide," she wrote. "And a story, a novel even. Must get out SNAKE PIT. There is an increasing market for mental-hospital stuff. I am a fool if I don't relive, recreate it."

As at Smith, Plath was a "scholarship girl" at McLean, supported by the well-to-do novelist Olive Higgins Prouty, a forceful
and intelligent woman who had suffered her own nervous breakdown a quarter-century before. Talented and ambitious, Plath had
a knack for aligning herself with the best brains wherever she was,
and McLean was no exception. The psychiatrist with whom she
met every day was the aforementioned Ruth Tiffany Barnhouse, a
real New York Tiffany and a rare female doctor at McLean. Freud-
ians would call it a transference; whatever the case, Plath fell in
love with her doctor. In *The Bell Jar*, Plath invoked her *Mademoiselle* magazine training to describe "Dr. Gordon," as she called
Barnhouse in the book: "She wore a white blouse and a full skirt
gathered at the waist by a wide leather belt, and stylish, crescent-
shaped spectacles. This woman was a cross between Myrna Loy
and my mother," Plath concluded. Who could ask for anything
more?

Although Plath did provide vivid descriptions of life at McLean
in her letters, she rarely discussed her therapy. In one sense, there
was not a great deal to discuss. When Plath first arrived, Barnhouse
decided to supplement psychotherapy with insulin shock treatment, which not only failed to address the patient's acedia but also
caused her face to bloat up and bruise, spoiling her natural beauty
and compounding her crisis of self-doubt. Like most McLean patients, Plath was dosed up on the antipsychotic drug Thorazine,
which contributed to her affectless behavior. Months after arriving, her therapy was blocked. "I got her to draw things first, and
then I had gotten her to talk, which was already something," Barnhouse recalled. "But she had been in there for months, and Mrs.
Prouty was paying the bills—this was going on and on. She was totally depressed and she wasn't getting any better."

Mrs. Prouty was visiting Sylvia regularly, and she was becoming
quite impatient with McLean. In November, she wrote a letter to
director Franklin Wood threatening to stop paying for a treatment
regime—Prouty felt it was nontreatment—that seemed to be leading nowhere. Prouty herself had spent time at Silver Hill in Con-

necticut, a mental hospital with a more structured approach to mobilizing depressed patients, and she could not abide McLean's laissez-faire attitude. "I usually find Sylvia wandering listlessly up and down the corridor and when I leave she says she will do the same, as there is nothing else for her to do," Prouty complained in a letter to Wood. Indeed, McLean was notorious for failing to fill "the other 23 hours" of the day, meaning the hours when the patients were not receiving psychotherapy.*

Plath's story was approaching its climax. Barnhouse decided to gamble and proposed electroshock therapy to the young girl. The idea of shock therapy was plenty scary, but it was especially scary to Plath, who had suffered through several painful and impersonal shock sessions at the hands of Dr. Peter Thornton and then Kenneth Tillotson at Valley Head Hospital that summer. She had received no anesthesia for the treatments, and after being semi-electrocuted, she had been wheeled into an empty recovery room to cope with her trauma. "She was not properly protected against the results of the treatment," Prouty wrote to one of Plath's doctors, "which were so poorly given that the patient remembers the details with horror." Prouty was a meddler, but an informed meddler, and she voiced her opinion that the botched electroshock sessions had driven Sylvia to attempt suicide. Plath herself later described the "rather brief and traumatic experience of badly-given shock treatments" at Valley Head to a friend: "Pretty soon, the only doubt in my mind was the precise time and method of committing suicide." But Barnhouse promised to stay

---

*Here are the comments of a woman who spent almost two years in Codman House at McLean, starting in 1963, after a stay at the Menninger Clinic in Topeka, Kansas: "I always mentally compared McLean with Menninger, and Menninger was just marvelous, it was beautiful, the appointments were incredible, fantastic, and the whole philosophy between the two hospitals was so different. Menninger kept you busy every minute, from 8 A.M. until you went to bed, they had your day planned for you. Where McLean's idea was, well if you get up, that's fine, we'd like to have you dressed by 8:30 or 9, but there were no real attempts to move you. Menninger would have you up doing these god-awful chores, stacking wood, and carrying wood to the doctors' houses, which was probably better for us in the long run."

with Plath during the McLean sessions and managed to convince the young woman that this time the results would be different.

They were. On December 15, Plath received the first of two shock treatments. She regained her personality and composure so rapidly that she was able to spend Christmas at home. Prouty brought her a typewriter, and Plath resumed her erudite and chatty correspondences with friends: feeling better; the company is swell. She rejoiced in the high-minded company: a classmate from Smith, girls from Vassar, Radcliffe, and Cornell, "plus an atomic genius from M.I.T." The hospital officially discharged her in late January, and by February she was back at Smith. Five years later, Plath mentioned the treatments in her journal: "Why, after the 'amazingly short' three or so shock treatments did I rocket up-hill? Why did I feel I needed to be punished, to punish myself." Neither she nor Barnhouse could explain the miraculous turnabout. "I can't tell you what happened," Barnhouse said in a 1998 interview.

> The human mind is very complex. . . . That sounds obvious but people keep forgetting it. They think you just throw a little Prozac in here, and a little of something else in here, it'll do this, this and this. It's ridiculous.
>
> Nobody can explain why Sylvia got over her depression after one or two shock treatments. She just didn't want to have any more shock treatments, so she reorganized herself inside so she wouldn't have any more. I never saw it happen with anybody else, but I wouldn't be surprised if it did happen.

Most psychiatric hospitals still administer a milder form of shock treatment, more palatably rechristened "electroconvulsive therapy," to blocked patients. When it works, doctors are still at a loss to explain how.

Barnhouse and Plath continued to see each other long after their McLean encounter. When Plath lived in Boston in 1958 and 1959, she saw Barnhouse professionally, as often as once a week. To Plath's considerable chagrin, she often lacked the money to pay her therapist, who lowered her hourly rate to five dollars to accommodate the struggling young poet. On Plath's side, the transference held strong. She wrote often about her need to be "worthy" of Barnhouse's friendship. She idolized the older woman, who seemed to be successfully juggling her psychiatric career with a strong marriage in which she bore responsibility for the raising of three small children. (The marriage later broke up.) By contrast, Plath fretted constantly about her career and worried that having children with her poet husband, Ted Hughes, would impede her literary progress. Although Barnhouse probably would not have admitted it–she soured on both Plath and Hughes at the end of her life–the psychiatrist probably stuck with Sylvia, gratis, because she was flattered by the attentions of the rising literary star. "The paid business is (not silly) but irrelevant," Barnhouse wrote to Plath in 1962. "If I help you, it is my reward. I would love to have the dedication to RB. [Plath had talked about dedicating a book of poems to Barnhouse.] I have often thought, if I 'cure' no one else in my whole career, you are enough. I love you."

Their therapy sessions worked wonders for Plath. "Better than shock treatment," Plath wrote in her journal. To Plath's great satisfaction, Barnhouse gave her "permission" to hate her mother: "'I hate her, doctor.' So I feel terrific. In a smarmy matriarchy of togetherness it is hard to get a sanction to hate one's mother especially a sanction one believes in. I believe in RB's because she is a clever woman who knows her business and I admire her." A few months later Plath wrote: "RB has become my mother."

Plath and her husband moved to London in 1960. The therapy sessions ended, although Plath did telephone her old friend and mentor on rare occasions. In late 1962, Plath's marriage plunged into crisis; Hughes was having an affair. Sylvia wrote Barnhouse a despairing letter. To use contemporary jargon, Barnhouse was there for her; her own marriage had ended in divorce, and she offered Plath plenty of emotional support and tough, practical advice for dealing with wayward husbands. "Frankly, I am furious at Ted," Barnhouse announced in September 1962:

> Has he left you? OK, sad, tragic stupid, unfortunate, anxiety-provoking, BUT NOT THE END. There are other ways of life, which may or may not involve another man. . . . You help neither him nor yourself by going down in a whirlpool of HIS making. Decide what you will put up with and what you will not. Stick to it. Don't be anyone's doormat. Do your crying alone. . . .
>
> The psychiatric pitfall that I see is your succumbing to the unconscious temptation to repeat your mother's role—i.e., martyr at the hands of the brutal male. If he really needs a succession of two-dimensional bitchy fuckings, let him have it. Set your conditions (quietly, in your own mind). Get a good lawyer, make him feel the bit of responsibility for the children (BUT NOT FOR YOU) in his pocketbook. Stand back and be an old-fashioned lady. If he is a boor, throw him out. If you happen to want to go to bed with him, do.

Nine days later, Barnhouse was lecturing Plath on the importance of selecting a first-class nanny ("Get a really, really good one") to throw into the child-care breach and offering more, concrete suggestions on coping with her rapidly dissolving marriage.

> If you really mean it about separation and not liking him, I would advise going whole hog and getting a divorce. You can certainly get the goods on him now while he is in such a reckless mood. If you wait, until he finds out a) you're not as spineless as he thought and b) maybe he made a mistake and wants to wiggle in again, you'll have a much harder time getting the evidence. . . .
>
> The rest, you have said for yourself. Keep him out of your bed. In the U.S., if a woman sleeps with her husband after he has committed adultery, she can no longer sue him for divorce on those grounds as

her act of sleeping with him constitutes condoning his misdoing. That is the practical reason. The other reasons you already know.

Plath and Hughes formally separated the following month. Four months later, Plath committed suicide at the age of thirty.

∽

*In 1968, Anne Sexton got her wish, sort of. Like a bolt from the blue, Sex-*ton received an invitation to teach a poetry seminar at McLean:

> Dear Mrs. Sexton,
> During the past two months, I have been directing quite a small group of McLean patients who write. Some are quite talented; some of the poems, especially, are fascinating.
> I have heard you had, at one time, an interest in the writings of psychiatric patients; the patient who told me this is a great admirer of yours and suggested I invite you to address the group. I would like to amplify her suggestion to include a possible series of workshop or lecture meetings which you would lead. Your visit or visits would be immensely valuable to motivate as well as instruct the patients.
> Margaret Ball, Patients' Librarian

The librarian's proposal was well timed. Not only was Sexton still fascinated by McLean, but she had just befriended a young Philadelphia poet named C.K. Williams, who had been teaching poetry in a mental hospital. Williams was ghostwriting books for local psychiatrists and had started up a literary magazine edited by the disturbed patients of the Institute of the Pennsylvania Hospital. "The editorial meetings started becoming group therapy, and we started taking advantage of that," Williams remembers. The formal term the psychiatrists used to describe the patients' quasi-literary outpourings was "primary process thought." "The thing I found amusing was that the people who were most floridly psychotic would talk like geniuses but write very conservatively," Williams told me. "The rule seemed to be that the crazier you were the better you talked but the worse you wrote. This was the group I had told Anne about." Sexton was fascinated by Williams's experiment and anxious to replicate his work at McLean.

Still, she had her doubts. "Anne was quite agitated one day, and called and said she'd been asked to do a poetry workshop at McLean," recalls Ames. "She saw this as an enormous responsibility. 'What if they're suicidal?' she asked. 'What if I say something about a poem that sends them over the edge?'" Furthermore, except for a high school seminar she had arranged with a friend, Sexton had never taught before. The pair decided that Ames, an experienced social worker, would help her teach the seminars at McLean.

The seminar assembled every Tuesday evening in the hospital library. Typically, Sexton would read a few poems written by her contemporaries, such as Diane Wakoski, Frederick Seidel, Robert Bagg, and Aliki Barnstone. Discussion would range from highly agitated to desultory, depending upon the mix of student-patients in the room. Sexton would ask each participant to prepare one or more poems for the following session, which Margaret Ball would collect during the week. Ball then sent the poems to Sexton's Wellesley home, where she read them and prepared her comments for the next class.

Some of Sexton's initial trepidation about her new charges was confirmed. From week to week, there was no way of knowing which patients might show up for the seminar. Although some patients enjoyed privileges to meander around the hospital grounds or even take the subway into town, others emerged from maximum-security wards with aides, dubbed "angels," holding them gently by the wrist, meaning that the patient was on suicide watch. Some patients' conditions varied from hour to hour, not to mention day to day. A patient who wrote an excellent poem might then disappear for several weeks until his or her condition improved.

Robert Perkins, an author and documentary filmmaker now living in Cambridge, Massachusetts, described the seminar in his 1994 memoir *Talking to Angels:*

> While I was [at McLean] Anne Sexton taught a poetry-writing class. She would come every two weeks to meet with a small group of aspiring poets. It was as boring a two hours as any other, although some of the students were entertaining. These wackos would rise to their feet and make up their poems right there, often yelling them out loud. A chorus of nutcakes. Occasionally, Anne Sexton would speak, but more often she sat there with the rest of us and let events swirl around her. If people wanted to argue about poetry or about poems, that was fine with her. Most of us, and I was one, could barely raise our heads, let alone write poetry or find anything intelligent to say.

Eleanor Morris, then a young patient who had dropped out of Bryn Mawr several years before, preserves a different memory of the sessions with Sexton:

> I have a mental image of Anne leaning on something in the library, maybe a piano, and the rest of us sitting around in chairs. She assigned us exercises, and you had to read your own poetry, which took a lot of courage. What I remember most is the blue, blue eyes. Her eyes were a piece of hope for me to see every week, they were daring me to do something.

Ellen Ratner, who has channeled her intense energy into a successful career as a syndicated radio talk-show host and television commentator, now reflects cynically on the proceedings: "Frankly I couldn't care less about poetry but she was famous and I wanted to meet someone who was that well-known." Ratner called Sexton, who was often mistaken for a model or an actress, "Sexy Anne," and even questioned her motives for teaching the "loonies." Ratner remembers, "I said, 'Well, Sexy Anne, why are you doing this?' She replied that she wanted to 'give back,' this that and the other. I always had the impression that she was teaching us either as a way to gather more material for her poems or she was doing it for her biography, since her biographer [Ames] was in the room."

To be fair, there is no evidence that this suggestion is true. Sexton kept few notes of the sessions, and most of those were teaching guides for herself. She wrote only one poem, "Out at the Mental Hospital," about her experiences at McLean, and she never published it:

> *No one has been tamed out at McLean*
> *See how the machine man is pounding with his stick!*
> *Notice that the pole girl rides a noon plane*
> *over her lunch. The clock browses. It's sick . . .*
> . . .
> *Let us have pity,*
> *Let us have pity.*
> *Night comes on and the nurses offer up a pill*
> *while the stars in the sky burn like neon jacks.*

There was no shortage of breeding or brainpower in the Sexton seminars. Perkins sprang from one of Boston's venerable First Families; he had interrupted his studies at Harvard for a year to acquire his McLean "diploma." Morris was a collateral relative of Ralph Waldo Emerson and Frederick Law Olmsted. But Sexton's favorite student proved to be a young girl from Fort Smith, Arkansas: Eugenia Plunkett, who had suffered a nervous breakdown at Radcliffe College and checked into McLean.

Plunkett, an attractive and precocious high school poet, had been a patient at McLean for five years before meeting Sexton. The transition from Arkansas to Radcliffe and Cambridge of the 1960s had overwhelmed her. "She wasn't prepared for the transformation to Harvard," says her younger brother Robert, a businessman in Fort Smith. "Her grades had been straight A's beforehand, but the competition was pretty tough. She wanted to have more of a social life, but she didn't know how to proceed."

It may have been Plunkett who suggested that the patient librarian invite Sexton to teach at McLean. Although she made much of being shy, she sent Sexton some of her poems before the seminar began and emphasized that she was a big fan. In one note, she told Sexton, "I feel like your stringbean girl," a reference to a famous poem ("Little Girl, My Stringbean, My Lovely Woman") that Sexton had written on the occasion of her daughter Linda's eleventh birthday.

The two women corresponded between classes. Sexton gossiped about the other patients in the seminar and enjoyed sharing confidences with her young acolyte. When Plunkett announced that she had left her psychiatrist because he had divorced his wife and refused to embark on an affair with her, Sexton—no stranger to the temptations of the therapist's couch—reacted knowingly:

> He could have handled it better. Of course you felt rejected, but it seems too bad that you had to stop seeing him. One thing I'll say. All the psychiatrists I've seen have been crazy and yet I learn from them. From your description of him you certainly wouldn't want to be married to him, but I know the feeling better than you think.

Sexton offered heartfelt congratulations on Plunkett's success when she published poems in the *Hudson Review* and the *American Scholar* during the seminar. And she did not hesitate to criticize Plunkett's work more firmly than that of the other patients. Upon receiving one batch of Plunkett's poems, Sexton wrote her, "I find them quite different and not worth much bother on your part. . . . Frost once said a poem should be 'lively,' not personal. I say a poem should be personal—in the sense of somebody having really lived something they are writing about."

At other times, Sexton would proffer advice tempered by her own considerable self-doubt: "Your work is very accomplished.

You have tons of talent. Still, I feel you are holding something back, some emotions you don't dare speak of. Do you wish it that way, I wonder? And then again should you listen to me—the me who is known for spilling her guts? . . . I can't think rationally and you can. I envy that." Sexton said more than once that she "envied" Plunkett's abilities, and of course the young poet was duly flattered: "I was quite proud to hear you envy my poem—I hadn't expected that at all, and it is quite a flattering thing to know."

One of Plunkett's most harrowing and successful poems appeared in the *Hudson Review*. Entitled "Encounter, Psychiatric Institute," it took place at McLean:

> *That awful*
> *Anonymity.*
> *She smiled at me*
> *From her pinned-down, stretch-out position flat*
> *On the tilted stretcher two big men*
> *Were hustling down the stairs. "And whom have I*
> *To thank for care of me?" she seemed to say.*
> *She smiled at me. Dark red and bright red were*
> *The colors of her arm. Suddenly I knew she'd done that shredding.*
> *Dire, innocuous smile!*
> *That anonymity? All people, strange*
> *(Sudden, yet by an awful, slow degree*
> *I knew), could never get a small word in*
> *On her dark room, her razor, finger, arm,*
> *Or her blind soul presiding. "Hear ye!" she*
> *Said to the dark room of the world, alone.*
> *And later even, outside, like galaxies*
> *Of rocks—the stars—or animals—the dogs—*
> *All we could ever do was stand and stare.*
> *And there, the arm, bare. Like her own soul, bare.*
> *She smiles at me across the ribbons—flesh—*
> *That say, "I am alone—without a sound*

You talk, without a recognition see
The star, the animal, the blood of me."

In the summer of 1969, Plunkett returned to Arkansas, where she remained in touch with Sexton. In June, she announced that she had again been institutionalized; "No sweat, though, be out soon, I think." She described the experience of listening to Sexton's poetry/rock record, *Anne Sexton and Her Kind:* "I cried all the way through 'Her Kind.' . . . The music is haunting, but nothing to the words. Had to hold my aide's hand—she, poor kid, not having the faintest idea of what was going on."

That was the summer of the moon landing, and Plunkett sent Sexton a poem about the event. In her last letter to her former student, Sexton wrote, "I was pleased that you sent the poem to me although I didn't understand it. Your rhyming is very skillful, but I do hear you, Jeanie, I do hear you sing." Later that year, Plunkett published her only book of poetry, *If You Listen Quietly,* which included the poem "Fragment for Anne." Sixteen years later, after an adulthood beset with psychological and physical disorders, she died of a neurological seizure in Fort Smith at the age of fifty-three.

How good were the other students' poems? A few of them were very good and were eventually published. Most of the poems were student quality, some good enough to print in the hospital newsletter. And some were just blots, words scrawled on paper by men and women shocked into the verges of catatonia.

One anonymous patient satirized his mental predicament:

> *Once I could*
> *and now I can't*
> *Write poetry*
> *I merely rant*

Sexton believed in encouraging all of her McLean students. When the late journalist John Swan wrote a poem called "Kids," describing his feelings for the his two young daughters, Sexton handed back his work with "GOOD" swathed across the page in capital letters. When she read this fragment of Swan's,

> *This last time*
> *When the children were told I was off*
> *For another rest . . .*
> *Lynn cried quietly . . .*
> *Her real cry.*

Sexton responded, "Powerful—maybe better than anything Lowell or Sexton has done on the subject." The praise was real, and her comment anything but casual. At the time, Sexton perceived Lowell as an important competitor, and both poets had trouble expressing affection for their children in their poems.

At one point, Plunkett chided Sexton for being too solicitous of her students' feelings. "You seem afraid to discourage anybody."

In a letter, Sexton responded, "You are right. I don't like to discourage anyone at McLean. I feel that everyone has something to say and will perhaps, in time, have more important things to say. Poetry led me by the hand out of madness. I am hoping I can show others that route." But Plunkett's complaint wasn't quite true. When Sexton sensed that one of her students could take constructive criticism, she freely dished it out. She continually pressed one of her poets, who later published a small collection of his poems, to push himself beyond writing fragments and expand into poetical form. He sent her these lines from a poem called "Anticipating Sexton":

> *I thought her eyes were green*
> *before she came. . . . The scene*
> *was her with lanky bone*
> *and skirt above bare*

thigh past knee . . .
Exalted like a queen among sin
and those who only half dared to reach for help. But I believed
that anywhere she'd come would be where
all sorts of thoughts, ill-formed, might get conceived,
and come out twitching, perfect infants through the hair
I imagined she had never let them shave.
She seemed, before meeting, to be, in that way, say, brave.

She wrote back, "Good ending" and asked for "another verse about what she is like—however disappointing to me personally."

Perhaps better than Plunkett, Sexton understood how close to the precipice some of her students were standing. Three girls in East House produced a mimeographed book for Sexton, entitled: "Behind the Screen: Poems from the Maximum Security Hall." Several were on suicide watch and wrote about it. One not untypical fragment:

> *(Half the skill of succeeding at suicide*
> *Comes with having a decent knife.)*

"The needs are so immense at McLean," Sexton wrote halfway through the seminar. "And although I try to meet them I generally fail."

In the spring of 1969, conflicting commitments started pulling Sexton away from the McLean seminar. She taught her last class in June. She corresponded with several of the patients for a few years after the class. Although she eventually lost touch with them, several followed her high-profile career in the newspapers and magazines.

Perhaps inevitably, the intensely self-critical and depressive Sexton viewed the seminar as a failure. In December 1973, she gathered some of the McLean poems and notes into a manila folder and scrawled a note in felt-tipped pen on the outside cover: "First teachings of creative writing—1969 (very difficult due to my insufficient knowledge of handling groups and the fact that the group was constantly changing and the aides were easily mixed up with the poets—Decide more commitment on the part of the poet is needed for me to be able to teach well.")

Whatever her misgivings, the McLean seminars did give Sexton the confidence to press forward with teaching. One of the McLean students organized a weekly seminar for his Boston-area Oberlin classmates at Sexton's home. Then Sexton arranged a faculty appointment at Boston University, where, in the 1970s, her poetry seminars achieved the same mythic cachet accorded to Lowell's classes in the 1960s.

The McLean students seemed to love Sexton, for her celebrity, for her own struggles with mental illness, and for the effort she invested in the course. Margaret Ball, who sent Sexton periodic updates on the patients' lives between the seminars, informed her more than once that her works were stolen more than any other author's: "'All My Pretty Ones' (replacement volume 4) lasted 1 week on the shelf before stolen. . . . It's their highest compliment, because usually they're so honest."

Robert Perkins, who remembers Sexton as "very pretty and very nervous," wrote that "I've since come to appreciate how difficult it must have been for Anne Sexton to come back to the hospital and deal with a group of loonies. She had been there herself. Maybe she felt she could help one of us. Maybe she did."

☙

In 1973, Sexton's awful wish was finally granted in full; she was admitted to McLean as a patient for five days of psychiatric examination. The grim "Patients' Property Form" is one of the few documents remaining from this visit, detailing that Sexton surrendered her nine credit cards—one from the Algonquin Hotel—and $220 in cash and traveler's checks ($5 in dimes, presumably for parking meters) on August 2 and reclaimed her effects on August 7.

Sexton's former student Eleanor Morris met her teacher unexpectedly in the North Belknap medium-security hall. "She remembered me from the seminar, but we didn't talk much," Morris recalls. "She looked so awful. . . . my heart went out to her." Here was the terrible leveling of mental illness; Sexton, the elegant, chain-smoking, Pulitzer Prize winner cast adrift among her student-patients on the desperate ocean of unhappiness. Sexton was just one year away from her own suicide, firmly embarked upon her *Awful Rowing Towards God,* the title of her last collection of poems.

Morris still remembers her clock radio waking her on Saturday, October 5, 1974. A newsreader announced that the poet Anne Sexton had died. "It just said she had died, but I knew she had committed suicide, and I spent the whole morning crying," Morris says.

Morris still has a copy of a book of poems that Sexton gave her after one of the seminars, a 1966 collection called *Live or Die.* In the flyleaf, Sexton wrote: "My directive is LIVE—to Ellie."

Eleanor Morris is living and writing poetry in Concord, Massachusetts.

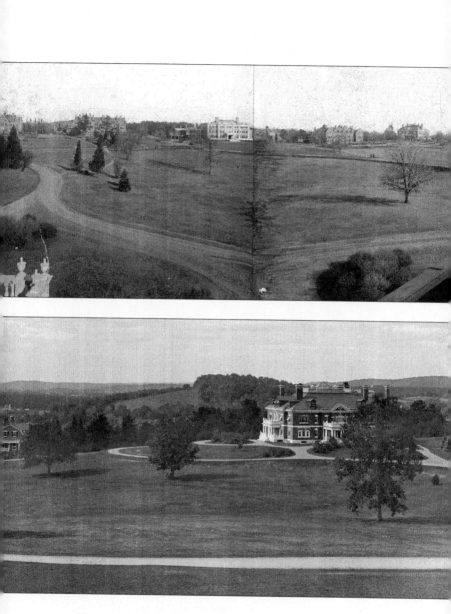

Views of the McLean Hospital grounds, 1900.
Credit: McLean Hospital.

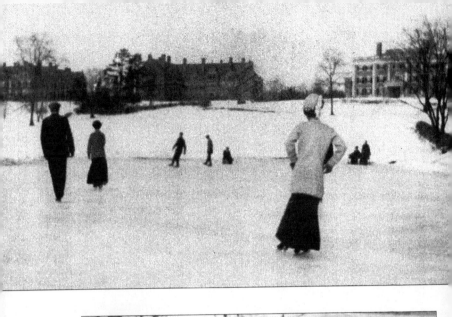

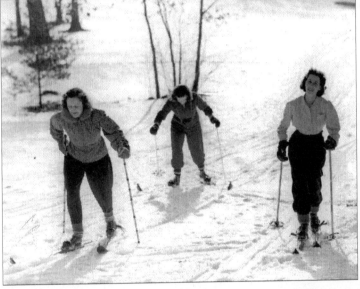

In these pictures taken during the late 1930s and early 1940s, nurses and aides skate on the "Bowl," a concave expanse of lawn in front of the administration building; ski in the woods surrounding the hospital; and play croquet, tennis, and golf. Patients took part in these activities though they were never photographed for reasons of privacy.
Credit: McLean Hospital.

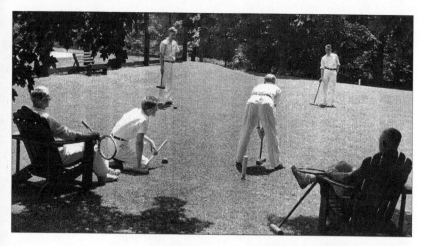

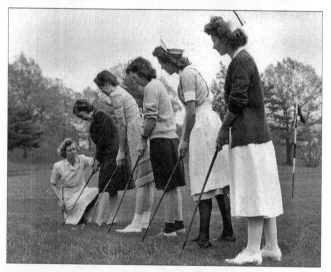

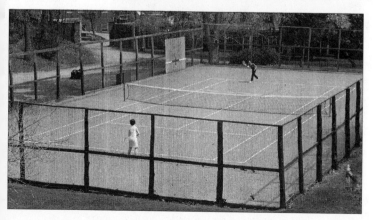

Horse and carriage, used to take patients on outings and visits, 1920. *Credit:* McLean Hospital.

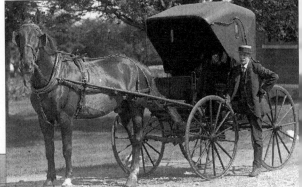

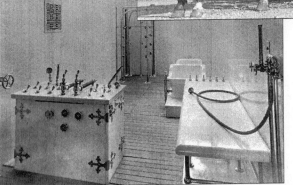

A hydriatic suite where nurses and aides administered the many different forms of hydrotherapy. *Credit:* McLean Hospital.

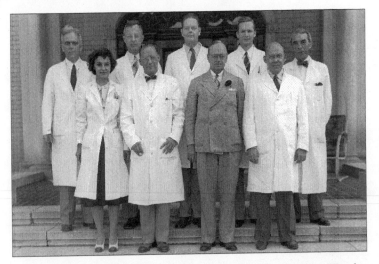

A photo of the McLean medical staff in 1945. Director Franklin Wood stands in the front row, center, in a gray suit wearing his trademark red carnation. At his right is psychiatrist-in-chief Kenneth Tillotson, who later became embroiled in an opéra bouffe sex scandal involving a McLean nurse. *Credit:* McLean Hospital.

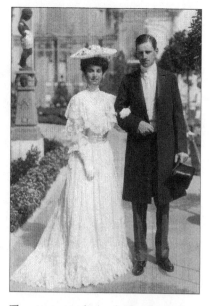

The star-crossed couple Stanley and Katharine McCormick, on their wedding day, in 1904, in Switzerland. Stanley, an heir to the International Harvester fortune, lived at McLean for two years and eventually moved his doctors and nurses west to a family estate in Santa Barbara. *Credit:* State Historical Society of Wisconsin.

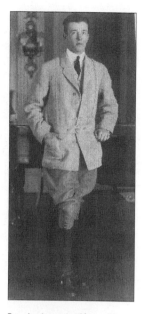

Louis Agassiz Shaw II, the wealthy society "novelist" who never stood trial for strangling his maid at his mansion in 1964. Instead, his lawyer won him a lifetime of luxurious living at McLean. *Credit: Boston Globe.*

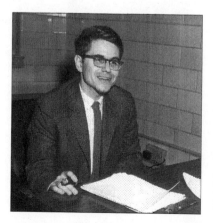

Dr. Harvey Shein, the brilliant young director of residency training whose suicide traumatized the hospital in 1974. *Credit:* McLean Hospital.

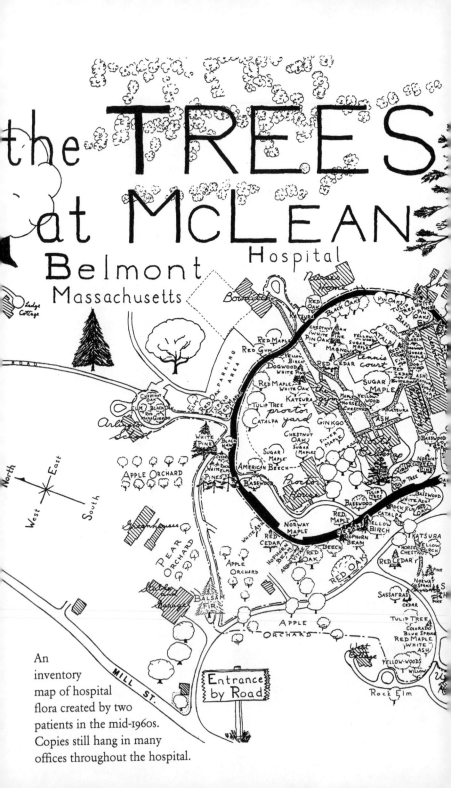

the TREES at McLEAN Hospital

Belmont Massachusetts

An
inventory
map of hospital
flora created by two
patients in the mid-1960s.
Copies still hang in many
offices throughout the hospital.

KEY
to the map

〜 9/10 mile loop, walk along road

≈ paths and walks

〜 other roads

☐ enclosed areas

▨ buildings

boundary, when unaccompanied freedom of the grounds is prescribed by a physician

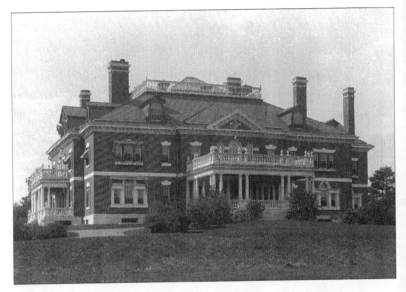

Upham Memorial Hall, the magnificent "Harvard Club" of McLean. At one time, Harvard graduates supposedly occupied each of its sumptuous corner suites. *Credit:* McLean Hospital.

Staying On

THE ELDERS FROM

PLANET UPHAM

When people came out here with major mental illness, the problem was, they just stayed. McLean did have a lot of long-term patients, so if somebody came out, the family would just say good-bye.

Dr. Stephen Washburn

*Psychiatrists hardly ever use the word "cure." They try to help pa-*tients, many of whom become "clear," successfully freeing their minds from the shackles of anxiety, depression, or more severe mental illness. But the profession's wellness model is like that of oncology. To be cancer-free or mentally healthy is to be in the happy state of remission. But many patients never get there. Some patients never improve or improve only marginally, and in the McLean of the not-too-distant past, that meant they never left the hospital.

A young female social worker who worked in McLean's children's program during the 1980s told me about a group of particularly old patients whom the children called the "elders." Ageless, wraithlike, oddly spectral, they were both scary to the children and also objects of infant mockery. They were quite literally a dying breed. They lived in the old style, in comfortably furnished single rooms. They had bookcases, attractive bedspreads, and furniture brought from home. Of course, they *were* home. Some of them had called McLean home for decades.

One of the white-haired old men was Louis Agassiz Shaw, a venerable Brahmin who had spent more than twenty years at McLean and was soon to be shipped off to a North Shore nursing home to die. A descendant of both Robert Gould Shaw, the heroic Civil War captain played by Matthew Broderick in the movie *Glory,* and of Louis Agassiz, the Swiss-born Harvard zoologist who revolutionized the study of biology, Shaw started off in the right direction.* He attended Noble and Greenough School, where he made his mark as a student poet. From Nobles, as it is called, Shaw proceeded to Harvard, where he joined the Porcellian Club, a watering hole for aristocratic "legacies": boys whose

---

*Because of the Boston aristocracy's penchant for marrying "cousins"—usually distant relatives—the name Louis Agassiz Shaw is less rare than one might think. For instance, there was a Harvard medical professor named Louis Agassiz Shaw who was arrested in 1927 for operating a still out of his "palatial home on 6 Marlboro Street in the Back Bay," according to the *Boston Globe.* Like my Louis, he too graduated from Noble and Greenough School and Harvard, although unlike his McLean namesake, this man made a genuine contribution to society: Professor Shaw invented the iron lung.

The name Louis Agassiz Shaw also crops up in Sylvia Plath's journal in her description of an April 1959 visit to a Beacon Hill neighbor: "She came from a family of Shaws, her son married a Shaw (no relation) and her daughter, (about 45?) had a young man, also a Shaw, Louis Agassiz Shaw, (Junior), and her daughter-in-law's uncle, or father, was also, oddly enough, named Louis Agassiz Shaw." One of these men must have been my Louis; the Harvard professor and inventor of the iron lung had been dead for nineteen years.

fathers and often grandfathers and beyond had attended the college. In his senior year, 1929, Shaw published a novel, *Pavement*,
under the pen name Louis Second. (His full name was Louis Agassiz Shaw II.) The book is almost unreadable and was probably
printed at Louis's expense; there is no trace of it in the *Literary Di-
gest*, which reviewed most novels of the time.* Ten years after graduating, and at five year intervals afterwards, Shaw dutifully, if
laconically, reported to his Harvard classmates on his activities:
"Engaged in writing for various publications and anthologies.
. . . on office staff of Citizens' Committee of U.S.O. . . . member,
St. Botolph, Somerset and Myopia Hunt Clubs." He often rode to
Myopia, an exclusive polo club, along bridle paths that linked his
fifteen-room Topsfield mansion with the club and with the neighboring estate of General George Patton. Twenty-five years out of
college, he had little to show for himself, especially when compared with Harvard graduates climbing the ladders of business,
government, and the arts.

Louis had two distinguishing characteristics: He was eccentric,
and he was a snob. In the entrance hall to his mansion, Shaw used
a plaster cast of his own foot to collect visitors' calling cards instead of the customary silver tray. He also kept a copy of the Social Register next to his telephone and instructed domestics not to
accept calls from men and women not listed there. When Shaw
had his house painted, he insisted that the workmen place large
metal trays under their scaffolding to ensure that no drips or
scrapings fell into his garden. He arranged for frequent and costly
repairs to the mansion and always waited a year before paying the
"tradesmen." A Nobles classmate, the landscape architect Sidney
Nichols Shurcliff, recalls that Louis publicly humiliated him for

---

*Although there is of course the odd nugget to entice serious Shavians. Louis would later tell
his McLean caretakers that he had been mistreated as a child, locked in closets when he was
bad, and so on. In *Pavement*, his protagonist, the wealthy, aspiring flapper Kit, serves up this
grim condemnation of the wonder years: "Most childhood is oppression and suppression and
depression, however much poets sing and grandparents cry over their silver pushers."

accepting a glass of cool lemonade from Louis's maid in the servants' quarters one scorching summer day.

Moving into his fifties, Louis was leading the not altogether unusual life of the educated, ineffectual, Boston twit. He rode to the hunt. He appeared at his clubs. In the Thirty-fifth Anniversary Report to his Harvard classmates, he provided no details of his life other than his home address in Topsfield, Massachusetts—incorrectly, as it turned out. In fact, he had taken up residence at McLean Hospital.

Shaw was in McLean because he had killed someone. "Cousin Louis did something that was highly inappropriate," is how his relative Parkman "Parky" Shaw, a longtime pillar of the Beacon Hill Civic Association, put it to me. When we first discussed Louis, Parkman and I experienced a classic Boston misunderstanding. "He's the one in the Robert Lowell poem," I said, meaning that Louis was clearly "Bobbie, Porcellian '29" in the famous poem "Waking in the Blue." "No, that's *Robert Gould* Shaw," Parkman corrected me. But we were talking about different Lowell poems; Parkman meant Lowell's memorably dispiriting "For the Union Dead," which evokes the bitter sacrifice of Robert Shaw's "bell-cheeked Negro infantry" parading across the Boston Common just two months before their bodies, and Shaw's, would be tossed into a mass grave after their suicidal attack on Fort Wagner, South Carolina. Once we cleared that up, we moved on to discuss Louis's "highly inappropriate" action: He had strangled his fifty-six-year-old Irish maid, Delia Holland, one night inside his sprawling mansion. According to the newspapers, Louis told police that Holland had been planning to kill *him* by turning on "secret gas jets" in his bedroom. Here is an account by the arresting officer, David Moran, of Louis's last night of freedom:

> I pushed through the second door. . . . the room was a library. Stacks of books wall-to-wall and floor-to-ceiling. Books.
>
> And a man in an armchair staring at me.

At the opposite end of the room was a fiftyish guy seated calmly in a stuffed chair. I figured it had to be the owner, Shaw. Amazingly, he showed no observable reaction to a state trooper stalking into his study with a long-barreled thirty-eight for a calling card. What bothered me even more was his calm demeanor when a dead body lay outside his door. . . .

I leveled my gun on him. It wouldn't have taken too belligerent a move under the [lap robe that Louis was wearing] for me to react. Finally, he acknowledged my arrival. But his look was as if I'd just tracked mud on his Persian carpet.

"And just who might you be?" His tone suggested that I'd also interrupted his morning meditation.

"State Police," I responded automatically. Taking a long shot, I blurted, "Why'd you kill her?"

"She was bothering me. Made too much noise!" he answered sedately. "I *told* her to stop."

Shurcliff reported that Louis killed Delia—the same maid who had been upbraided for serving him lemonade in the pantry—because she threatened to resign. In a self-published memoir, Shurcliff, a landscaper to the rich and famous, wrote that Louis "flew into a rage and effected her immediate resignation by choking her to death!"

Whatever the motive, the crime heaped shame upon the venerable Shaw family. "It was on the front pages of everything," Parkman Shaw lamented to me. Indeed it was. "Bay State Scion Admits Strangling His Maid," barked the *New York Herald*. "Louis Shaw Second Held in Strangle Death," cried the *Boston Globe*. The press had a field day. No story failed to mention Shaw's Harvard degree, his dilettante's lifestyle—he is alternately described as a "wealthy retired writer," "a mystery writer," a "country squire," and a "part-time author"—and his esteemed antecedents. Old Boston still remembers that Louis's father, Robert Gould Shaw II, had married Nancy Langhorne, who later became "the nutty Lady

Astor." The former Mrs. Shaw went on to marry Lord Astor and became a champion of social reform and "Tory democracy" (and, more disturbingly, of pro-Nazi sentiment) in midcentury England. She was also the first woman to win election to Parliament. At McLean, Shaw bruited to one and all that he was "related to the Astors," which, strictly speaking, he was not. Louis was the only child of his father's second marriage.

Louis had plenty of money, and he hired a deft, Harvard-trained lawyer who just happened to be a distant cousin, James Barr Ames of the white-shoe law firm Ropes and Gray. At his arraignment in Salem District Court, it emerged that Louis had been seeing a psychiatrist for more than ten years, and he tried to pick a fight with the clerk who read out the criminal charge. Louis never came to trial. Ames had him committed first to the state asylum at Bridgewater and then to the far more comfortable and familiar surroundings at McLean. "I don't believe cousin Louis was ever indicted," says Parkman, whose memory on this point of family lore proves to be quite precise. "He was remanded to Bridgewater State Hospital for the Criminally Insane, and then some time later he graduated to the McLean hospital where he was well liked and well respected."*

After a stint on Bowditch Hall, where Robert Lowell immortalized him as "Bobbie," Louis transferred to Upham Memorial, affectionately known as the "Harvard Club" because at one time, each of its majestic corner suites was said to have been occupied

---

*Louis wrote letters from Bridgewater to his friend Jonathan Bayliss, complaining about the "hellhole" of public accommodations: "This is an impossible place to be because the other inmates are so far gone. . . . Loud music blares all day. It is unbelievably terrible. . . . There are fifty-five other inmates in this room and except for two or three they are all looney." His lawyer held out hope for a transfer; "I'm hoping and praying it will be McLean's," Louis wrote. "So many people . . . tell me how their nephews or cousins or best friends have been there."

Once in Belmont, Louis waxes confident that the legal wizardry that kept him out of jail will soon free him: "It is quite likely that I may be home during the summer. This means that I shall be well enough (it is hoped) so that I can stand trial. The lawyer tells me that this will just be a formality and I will be acquitted and go home."

by a graduate of Harvard College. Indeed, when Louis arrived on Upham, there was no shortage of well-bred ladies and gentlemen to greet him. He must have felt right at home.

⚬

When they first committed themselves to the Belmont move in the 1880s, the McLean trustees approved construction of only two buildings: Belknap House, a combined office and residence space for thirty women, and Appleton, a residential ward for eight female patients. More or less out of the blue, George Phineas Upham, a partner in the merchant banking firm of Upham, Appleton, and Company, approached the board and offered to finance a third building as a memorial to his son, George Phineas Jr. A graduate of Harvard like his father, the young man had joined the family business but died unexpectedly at age thirty-two. Whereas the trustees had been using the leading institutional architects of the day, Upham insisted upon using his personal architect, William Peters, who had designed many a splendid residence in Boston's Back Bay. The resulting hall, Upham Memorial, was and is by far the most grandiose structure on the McLean campus. Sitting across the vast, grassy bowl from the rest of the hospital, Upham is a lavish, sprawling brick colonial pile larger than many hotels—and intended to house just nine male patients. (Women lived there, starting in the 1960s.) The exterior is bright red pressed Somerville brick trimmed with white Georgia marble. The foundation ("underpinning") is "hammered Troy Granite," according to the announcement of its completion; the roof is covered with "dark Eastern slate." The ground floor had two grand, open hallways, each featuring a sweeping, carved wooden staircase; the dining room; and four suites, each with fireplace and private toilet and bath. Writing for the *American Journal of Insanity,* Dr. Henry Hurd picked up the description:

There are two suites on the westerly side of the house which have an outlook towards the valley of the Charles. A short corridor leads from the rear hall past the serving room and adjoining the dining room, to an exit upon a terrace at the northwest corner of the house, and to the grounds in the rear.

The second floor, with its five suites, corresponding closely with those on the first floor, has also a billiard and smoking room over the dining room. All the rooms have fireplaces, ample closet room, etc., and a lobby intervening between them and the adjoining hall, so that the patient may have extreme quietude and seclusion from others when desired, or a disturbed patient may not annoy others.

The attic contains rooms for nurses. . . . There are also rooms for a cook and a housemaid.

Hurd neglected to mention the basement, with its large kitchen, pantry, storeroom, and sitting-room and dining room for the nursing staff. The basement also had "a special arrangement for Turkish and plunge baths, etc.," including three rooms and a dressing room, according to the hospital's annual report.

Geography isolated Upham. Because the grassy bowl—which doubled as the final fairway and hole in McLean's small-scale golf course—dipped about forty feet below ground level, no tunnels could be built connecting Upham to the rest of the campus. Upham had its own kitchens and functioned quite autonomously when winter snowstorms prevented staff and patients from entering or leaving the building. In McLean's modern era, as fees shot up and hospital stays became shorter and shorter, Upham resembled its own planet, populated by wealthy, chronic, long-term patients impervious to or uninterested in restorative therapy, who would live out their days wandering the corridors of George P. Upham's magnificent memorial to his son.

In the 1950s and 1960s, just when Alfred Stanton was trying to get the hospital moving again, Upham became a classic "back ward," a dumping ground for chronically ill, elderly patients—practically all of them rich—whose families had cut lifetime financial deals with the hospital. There was little incentive to "cure" the Uphamites because their families had paid good money never to see them again. "It was really a level four rest home," explains Dr. Bernard Yudowitz, who helped run Upham in the early 1970s. "These were people who were quite benign, very interesting and highly intelligent, who lived in their own world. These were the people who had been in the cottages in the pre-Stanton era," he says.

> They were the history of psychiatry, because whoever treated them went back to the late 1800s or the early 1900s. There were people there who had 200 shock treatments already, from the heyday of multiple shock treatments. There were people who had traveled the world to the most eminent psychiatrists of the day. They were the grand dames of McLean.

Dr. Richard Budson, who also worked on Upham, remembers the hall somewhat differently. As a young resident, he was startled by McLean's indifference to the mental health of this vestigial population:

> The patients were all obviously from very wealthy families, and the nursing staff treated them in the most patronizing way, as if they were quasi-incompetent, rich wealthy hand-me-downs. Their job was to give the patients elegant, comfortable custodial care that kept the families happy. Nobody did a damned thing with these patients. The view was that if the status quo was disrupted, all hell would break loose because they were potentially dangerous.

For many years, Upham was the ward that time forgot. There was a huge fir tree in front of the hall, where the Christmas lights stayed up well into the spring. "We would have a hall meeting every week," Yudowitz says, "and the topic would be 'When are we going to take the Christmas tree lights down from the tree outside?' And it could never be resolved." In March, sometimes as late as April, a maintenance worker would make his way over to Upham with a ladder and take the lights down.

∞

Although the criminal justice system had transported Louis Shaw about fifty miles from his Topsfield mansion, he really had not traveled very far at all. Upham in the 1950s and 1960s resembled a private, Ivy League residential club more than the chronic schizophrenic ward of a mental hospital. Scofield Thayer had mailed out his 1927 Christmas cards from Upham. Carl Liebman, the wealthy, Yale-educated Man Who Knew Freud, was still there, along with a host of oddities from McLean's curio shop of the American aristocracy. There was a woman called "The Moth" because she had jumped out of the Massachusetts General Hospital tower building and lived. The hospital's best-known oddball patients, Henry and William Ziegel, lodged there, in separate suites and rarely on congenial terms. Henry, an erudite Harvard man given to barking, "Henry Ziegel! Harvard, Class of 1913! You can tell a Harvard man, but you can't tell him much!" at passers-by, uncharitably referred to William as "my idiot brother." A natty dresser, Henry was a published research chemist and received American Chemical Society periodicals at Upham, where they attracted plenty of comment. Deemed harmless, he was allowed to take the trolley into Cambridge to audit chemistry classes at Harvard. Inevitably, he would return to Belmont and announce that "Cambridge was on fire," news doubtless intended to cause great consternation at McLean. In shop, Henry also assembled clocks from old parts and offered them as gifts to his nurses and doctors in gratitude for their care. Several dozen rudimentary "Ziegel clocks" are gathering dust in New England homes; it would be a miracle of engineering if any were still working.

Another star in the Upham firmament was Frank Everett, a gentleman from Colorado. Everett, who had been hospitalized after threatening family members, was famous for being the only McLean patient whose name appeared on a Secret Service watch list. He had written a letter threatening the life of the president—no one remembers which one—and the hospital had to dial a certain number in Washington if Everett ever escaped. He did once escape, and the number was dialed—and then redialed shortly afterwards, when he was discovered hiding in the McLean cafeteria.

Everett was a great worrier, indeed a paranoid, who employed a younger, female patient as his "poison tester." Like many patients, he feared medications. Even among McLean old-timers, he was something of a world-class "med-tonguer," meaning that he could stash any number of pills in the back of his mouth and spit them out when the nurses averted their gaze. When the maid came to clean his room, dozens of pills would clatter up through the metal handle of the vacuum cleaner. "M&Ms, my dear, just M&Ms," he would mumble, as several days' worth of psychopharmaceuticals were sucked off his carpet. Two voices spoke to Frank Everett: the good "Lenore" advised him through his right ear, and the bad "Beasley" spoke to his left ear. When it came time to swallow medication, "Beasley" prevailed.

Eternal vigilance was the price of Everett's paranoia, and instead of sleeping on his bed, he often slept sitting upright in a rocking chair in the hall outside his room. One of his favorite companions was Upham's young psychiatrist-in-chief, Dr. Harvey Shein, whom he would allow to sit in his beloved rocker while the men shared a cigar and cracked jokes. "When Harvey died, Frank turned that chair to the wall and never sat in it again," a friend of Everett's told me.

∞

The same psychiatrist who visited McLean in the 1950s *and remarked* upon the hospital's "feudalistic" and "medievalistic" culture had this to say about the patients: "Most of the patients looked to me

like social rejects of a blunted sort mixed with annoying neurotics.
. . . because of the high rates and the luxuriousness of the place,
aristocratic clientele is found, consisting of patients whose families *don't want them to get really well* [emphasis added]."

So it was, for example, with Louis Agassiz Shaw. No one really
wanted him to get well. The state did not want him to regain his
sanity because then he would have to stand trial for murder. The
hospital had no particular stake in the matter; Shaw's lawyers paid
his bills on time, and he was generally harmless. As for many of
the "thoroughbred mental cases," life inside McLean offered
Louis much more than life outside. So for twenty-three years, with
occasional escorted day trips to his Topsfield mansion or group
outings to a North Shore beach, Louis called a book-lined suite in
Upham Hall home.

Louis dressed oddly. "He'd get all dressed up as a cavalry officer
with a cloak over his shoulder when he came out to see me," recalls his lawyer James Barr Ames. "He always wore crisp, white
shirts, and he would wear paper towels on the inside of his col-
lars," a McLean staffer remembers, "and he would constantly pull
at his collar during community meetings. He didn't like anything
tight around his neck." A curious tic for a man who had strangled
his maid.

Louis continued to be a tremendous snob. His preferred psychiatrist was his Harvard contemporary Dr. Vernon Williams,
himself something of an odd duck who lived in a bachelor's
boarding house on Beacon Hill. ("The story was that Vernon had
been sent to psychiatry so he wouldn't kill anybody in medicine,"
a colleague recalls. "And he always traveled by train because his
mother never allowed him to fly.") Whether or how Williams actually treated Louis, no one knows. Paul Dinsmore, the psychiatrist in charge of Upham for a portion of Louis's stay, remembers
the two men singing Episcopalian hymns together during therapy
sessions. Louis's favorite companion at Upham was a renowned
Harvard professor of Asian studies who had tried to commit suicide nineteen times. On the twentieth attempt, he succeeded.

"Louis never spoke to me after that," says the doctor in charge of the case. "His psychiatrist said, 'Louis is very angry with you because you let Mr. ——— die.' I could understand that."

In his late seventies, Louis Shaw was a pale shadow of the lunatic who once strangled his maid. Nurses could control him relatively easily. To the younger generation, "He was a wonderful, gentlemanly character," remembers William Shine, a ward aide at McLean in the late 1960s. "He was quite distinguished looking, with white-ish hair. He wandered the grounds, wearing an overcoat in the winter, a blazer in the summer. He never spoke to anybody." In the mid-1980s, McLean officials decided it was time to part company with Louis. "It was getting to the point where it was becoming very expensive to have him here," says Dr. Peter Choras.

> He needed a lot of nursing care, and maybe he would have to be moved out to a nursing home. So we went to the lawyers and we proposed a deal. We named a price, about $500,000, and we said we'd keep Louis for that price. If he died in a year, we'd make a lot of money, but if he lived ten years, we'd lose a lot of money. It seemed unorthodox, but they didn't bat an eyelash. They liked the idea, and they thought Louis would approve, since he liked to gamble.

This was precisely the kind of deal that had gone sour for McLean in the past. One family supposedly paid the hospital a lump sum of $25,000 after World War I to warehouse a wayward scion. The patient lived another fifty years, contributing to McLean's deficits over the years.

But Louis did not live another ten years. In accordance with their custodial agreement, McLean decided to place him in a North Shore nursing home, not far from his ancestral manse in Topsfield. Administrators made the decision, which, interestingly, Louis's psychiatrist (not the long departed Vernon Williams) opposed. Even though Louis had never discussed the events of April 7, 1964, with his latest analyst, the doctor worried about loosing

Louis on the world. Medicated with mood-stabilizing drugs, Louis presented a gentlemanly, raffish demeanor to the outside world. But his therapist had a hunch that he could turn violent, and his hunch proved right. In the nursing home, Louis tried to attack a nurse, feebly, but aggressively nonetheless. Shortly afterwards, he died in Manchester, Massachusetts, which had just voted to re-name itself Manchester-by-the-Sea, to remind the public of its by-gone renown as the "Newport of the North Shore." I think Louis would have approved.

The passing of the privileged "Bay State scion" who had made front-page news in 1964 went unremarked by either Boston news-paper. When he died, Louis left almost $4 million in assets. Two million went to charity, and the Topsfield mansion, worth about one million, was donated to the Catholic archdiocese of Boston. Harvard's Fogg Museum turned down his $300,000 art collection. To put it gently, Louis was no Scofield Thayer. The Raphael, the Michelangelo, and the Leonardo that Louis showed off to visitors were fakes. The Fogg did take a bronze sculpture of Charles VII (Louis thought it was Joan of Arc) and a donation of $150,000. The rest of the money went to nieces, nephews, former servants, and the lawyers. Over the years, McLean had been trying to wheedle some money out of Louis's estate to pay for the restoration of the Pleasant Street gatehouse, where he lived for a while. They did not get a dime.

About halfway through my work on McLean, I met Mark Robart, the hospital's director of social work, at a party. We discussed my interest in McLean's vestigial culture. He asked me what kinds of sources I was using to research my book. "People," I answered. Out of the blue, he suggested that I interview "Walter Paton," a seventy-seven-year-old man who had resided at McLean since 1948. Paton was genial, excessively shy, and well liked by his caretakers. Flashing his hesitant smile, he often muttered that "things are quite a bit different now at the hospital" or "things really changed when Dr. Stanton got here." There had been talk of preserving his memories in an oral history. Instead, I was allowed to interview him, on the condition that I promised not to reveal his identity.

Walter now lives in Appleton House, which has been converted into an unlocked residential facility. He is not strictly speaking a patient at McLean, although he is living on the campus in the care of McLean doctors, for the comparatively cheap price of $195 a day (the rate for an inpatient day is about $900). The doctor in charge explained to me that the Appleton residents are men and women who suffered from psychotic events in their past but are now in remission. With the help of drugs, they no longer have to live on a ward. On the other hand, although they are free to roam around the grounds, they do not have the life skills to function in everyday society. Their meals are prepared for them, but the patients participate communally in some chores, such as kitchen clean-up. In Walter's case, it seemed fair to conclude that he would never leave the hospital. "There were lots of attempts to move him off grounds, but they weren't successful," his social worker told me. "This had become his own small town. Walking around the grounds with him is like walking around with the elder of a village."

Walter proved to be eager for the interview, and he was unfailingly polite when we met. He was dressed casually, in an open shirt, yellow cardigan sweater, slacks, and sensible shoes. With his stooped gait and thin, pencil mustache he resembled the older Leo G. Carroll, star of the long-forgotten (but not by Walter, I suspect) television series *Topper*. As advertised, he was quite shy, and he did have some trouble speaking. He also had motor control problems with his hands and arms.

Like many old people, Walter had some firm memories about the past. He remembered Paul Howard, the doctor who had admitted him to McLean, and he could easily tick off the wards where he had lived: Proctor, North Belknap, Upham, and Hope Cottage; the latter two had been closed down during the 1990s, and his program had moved to Appleton. He made a point of noting that he had never been on Bowditch, for many years the men's locked unit.

Walter had been cued to my interest in the old McLean, and he did repeat his pet phrase, "things are quite a bit different now at the hospital." When he arrived in the late 1940s, "there was a work horse here in the garage, and two riding horses. Then there got to be so many cars around it got too dangerous to ride." He correctly noted that there had not been a security department when he came to the hospital and that the longtime food service workers had been sacked during a cost-cutting drive.

Walter well remembered that Franklin Wood used to live just down the hill, in a grand residence now slated for demolition to make way for the office park. "Wood was a medical doctor but not a psychiatrist," Walter said. "Dr. Stanton was a psychiatrist. He really changed things around." For example? "Well, they never needed a stoplight down on Mill Street before he came. Then they got all these cars. He built Hall-Mercer [the brutalist, concrete-block child and adolescent center]—as for that architecture, the less said the better. They had some adults in there at one point and they said it felt like a jail." I told him that Hall-Mercer, too, was slated for demolition. "I don't think people will miss it," he said with a slight smile.

I wanted to talk about Upham, but it was not clear whether I could ask after specific patients. (A McLean staffer sat in on our conversation.) I asked if he recalled "the man who knew Freud," and without naming him, Walter recited the career highlights of Carl Liebman: "There was a patient who had gone to Europe to see Dr. Freud. I don't know what good it did him. He liked to read German philosophy books. Goethe. He had a lobotomy. He came from New York. His family was in the brewing business."

When I mentioned that Carl had attended Yale, Walter quickly corrected me. "But only for two years—he always said that people should be paid to go there." Walter had a reflexive answer for people and events he did not recollect. When I inquired about Ray Charles playing the piano in the Upham sitting room or about other patients, he just smiled and said, "Oh, I missed that."

When I asked after his family, Walter said he had a sister in the Worcester area who had lived in a large house that she had recently sold. Her children had all grown up, and she had since moved into a smaller condominium. About a year and a half earlier, one of his nephews had come to visit him on Appleton. "He said that he'd be back, but I don't know when," Paton recounted. "He said he wanted to get to know me, but maybe he didn't want to get to know me that well."

Walter told me more than once that "psychiatry has improved a lot," but he didn't sound particularly sincere. How had it improved? There are "more meds than forty years ago. It's sort of encouraging and it's sort of disappointing." How is it disappointing, I asked? "It's a mixed bag," he answered, changing the subject.

Two weeks later, I saw the McLean staffer who had sat in on our conversation. We both agreed that the meeting had not yielded much. On the one hand, I felt I had failed to make a positive connection with Paton—psychotherapy is hard! On the other hand, I felt that her presence, which was probably necessary for legal reasons, had exacerbated an already awkward situation. What did she learn, I asked? She told me that while Walter and I had been speaking, she had been calculating the number of days he had spent at McLean and then multiplied that number by $195. Since 1948, give or take a few hundred thousand dollars—long-term discounts were common for good customers—the Paton family had spent $3.5 million to lodge Uncle Walter at McLean.

∞

Toward the end of the 1960s, *the character of Upham gradually began* to change. In 1966, the patients must have been surprised to see a rare black face at their morning meetings; the great blues singer Ray Charles, then thirty-five years old, came onto the hall for a week-long "observational" visit.

Charles was on Upham not by the grace of a well-invested trust fund but by the grace of a broad-minded federal judge. A year earlier, customs agents at Logan Airport had busted Charles for possession of heroin and marijuana when he landed in Boston at 3 A.M. after a private plane flight from Canada. The blind singer's lawyers managed to delay sentencing for a year, and when the case came before Judge Charles Wyzanski, he offered Charles an alluring deal: four years' probation if the defendant agreed to check into McLean every six months for observation and if he tested negative for drugs. Charles described his first visit to Upham in his 1978 autobiography *Brother Ray*:

I went to sleep at about eight. At midnight I woke up to go to the toilet, and I was freezing to death. Godamn, it's cold in here. Can't understand it. Don't these people care about heat? I wondered. So I put on my robe and tiptoed out to the hall. Man, it was warm as toast out there—comfortable and cozy as it could be.

I knew what they were up to. When you're withdrawing from drugs, coldness quickens your sickness. You'll probably have chills when the temperature is normal, but when it's really cold, you suffer something awful. They wanted to see how bad I'd start shaking.

I called for the head nurse.

"Look mama," I said. "I'm not blaming you. I know you don't make the rules. But sweetheart, if I catch pneumonia, I'm gonna sue this place so bad that everyone here is gonna be working for me. I'm gonna own this joint. Got it?"

Five minutes later warm air was flowing through the ducts and I was snuggled back in bed.

There was a piano in Upham's huge, ground-floor living room, and Charles gave impromptu concerts for his hall mates. He reported that he played with "a classical cat, who could really wail." "The nicest part was meeting one of the nurses who I got next to a little later on," he added. Charles and the nurse remained an item during his subsequent visits to McLean, where he never tested positive for drugs.

Another nonstandard patient arrived on Upham in the early 1970s: Joan Tunney Wilkinson, daughter of the famous boxer Gene Tunney and sister of then-senator John Tunney. Wilkinson—young, beautiful, and well connected—had transferred into McLean from Broadmoor psychiatric prison in England.

According to press reports, Wilkinson "attacked her husband with a chopper" on Easter Sunday, 1970, in their home in Chenies, Buckinghamshire, a small village thirty miles from London. Although various insinuations were made concerning the couple's "hippy" lifestyle, no motive was ever adduced. Wilkinson's lawyers explained that she had suffered from schizophrenia for nine years, which won her admission to Broadmoor and eventually to McLean, where she could be closer to her family. At McLean, Wilkinson befriended a black cat named Felina and came under the sway of the Christian revival group The Way. She became a Bible-thumping companion of fellow murderer Louis Agassiz Shaw. At hall meetings, where Frank Everett would sometimes utter random cries of "Germs!" and "Pestilence!" Wilkinson was wont to say, "Louis, we must confess our sins." His inevitable answer: "Oh, Joan, no." If Louis ever confessed, he saved it for the confessional.

Around the time Wilkinson checked in, young people—*really* young people—started appearing on Upham. McLean had set up an adolescent treatment unit in the basement of the hall, and for the first time sixteen- and seventeen-year-old patients were roaming the same corridors as Liebman, Shaw, and the Ziegel brothers. The young patients, mostly boys, were disturbed, disturbing, disruptive, and even destructive. One boy put his hand through a screen that was supposedly designed to handle a 2,000-pound blow. Others knocked down the plaster flowers that adorned the light fixtures on the ground floor. Walter Paton recalled that one boy broke into the medication cabinet and assaulted a nurse who tried to stop him, breaking her glasses. The trashing of Upham had begun.

By the time I arranged a visit in April 2000, Upham was a disaster area. I remember Roberta Shaw, at that time McLean's director of public affairs, a somewhat abashed security guard, and myself standing on the second floor shoe-deep in plaster fragments, paint chips, feathers, and pigeon droppings, staring up at the once-magnificent atrium skylight that channeled sun down into the building's entry foyer. As part of its general downsizing, McLean had abandoned Upham a couple of years previously, partly because the hospital no longer needed the space and partly because Upham was not connected to the other buildings by Olmsted's tunnel system and thus was less convenient to maintain. Once the equivalent of a luxury hotel with nine superbly appointed suites, Upham had been fricasseed into ever-shrinking quadrants of offices and bedrooms over the years. Just before it was closed, Upham was a "gap sleeper," or temporary shelter for homeless men and women who drifted into McLean during the winter. Locked and abandoned after that, it had become a home for pigeons and mice and was awaiting the restoration efforts of the Northland Development Corporation, which planned to convert the stately mansion into five separate town houses, each priced at $600,000.

The security guard had reason to be abashed. Upham had not only been left to the elements; it had also been robbed and vandalized. An antiques thief had joined McLean's security force and systematically stripped Upham of valuable furnishings, mostly carved wooden mantelpieces, picture frames, and sconces. The Belmont police found fingerprints on a shard of mirror cast into the nearby forest, and the robber was eventually nabbed at a western Massachusetts antiques fair. McLean had managed to keep the embarrassing incident more or less under wraps. Under siege from thievery, pigeons, rodents, and the ravages of time, not much remained of the stately interior of McLean's magnificent "Harvard Club" except for the portrait of young George Phineas Upham Jr. hanging above the fireplace in the ground-floor salon.

Diagnosis

"HIPPIEPHRENIA"

It was by no means easy for us to decide when someone
had crossed the border from hippie to hippiephrenia.

Dr. Alan Stone

During his first major concert tour in 1969, James Taylor used to
introduce his song "Knockin' 'Round the Zoo" with a few words
about his stay in Belmont. "Here's a tune I wrote at McLean to
make a million bucks," he told one youthful audience. "McLean,
that's a mental hospital–O.K., anybody here from McLean? Let's
hear it for McLean." Few people clapped, of course, because very
few young people had spent time in mental institutions. But Taylor, then sporting a shoulder-length mop of dark, grimy hair,
would grin sheepishly at the light smattering of applause and proceed with his cryptic paean to his nine-month stay in the "zoo":

There's bars on all the windows and they're
counting up the spoons
And if I'm feeling edgy, there's a chick who's paid to be my slave
But she'll hit me with a needle if she thinks I'm trying to misbehave.

For a mellower, preppy cohort of the 1960s generation, the soft-singing Taylor siblings—James, his talented brother Livingston, and the singer always known as Sister Kate—put McLean on the map. "For the Taylors," *Time* magazine noted sardonically in a 1971 cover story on James, "the McLean experience would soon become what Harvard is for the Saltonstalls—something of a family tradition." A washout at tradition-bound Milton Academy, James thrived at McLean's newly opened Arlington School. "We didn't have that jive nothingness that pushes most kids through high school," he said. "You can't tell a whole bunch of potential suicides that they have to have a high school diploma." The product of a liberal, moneyed household, Taylor relished what he saw as the reassuring structure of the typical McLean day: "Above all, the day was planned for me there, and I began to have a sense of time and structure, like canals and railroad tracks." Taylor never claimed that McLean "cured" him—less than three years after "escaping" from the hospital, he found himself addicted to heroin and checked in to the more bucolic, twenty-three-bed Austen Riggs sanitarium in Stockbridge, Massachusetts—but it enabled him to establish a modus vivendi with the modern world. He and his sister Kate both have homes on Martha's Vineyard, and both have compared the island's laid-back pace to the asylum of McLean. "It was a pretty slow pace," Kate recalls. "Very slow. No pressure. And that continues for me, living on Martha's Vineyard, out here at the end of the trail" James now calls his McLean time

a lifesaver. I think it was a lifesaver. I've always thought of it like a pardon, or like a reprieve, with a sort of medical stamp of approval. Once I got there, my main concern was that they wouldn't let me stay, that they'd find out that I wasn't a serious case, that my bed might be needed by someone more worthy. I didn't want to be turned out of the place. I didn't want to go back to the life that I had been unable to lead.

Although James wrote his first two songs while still a patient in 1965, his path to success ran through New York City and then London, where he met the Beatles' producer Peter Asher, who fine-tuned the Taylor sound for the Apple label. (James's "escape" from McLean is still the subject of legend. Because he had committed himself voluntarily, he could not escape. He did, however, bolt for Manhattan without signing the customary "three-day," the required three days' notice before checking oneself out.) But Kate and subsequently Livingston launched their careers at McLean. Searching for therapies that might connect with their music-addled, alienated charges, McLean hired a young rock musician named Paul Roberts to conduct music therapy classes. Roberts had studied psychology at Brandeis and tried to play music on the wards at Metropolitan State, where he had gone to work as an aide to avoid the Vietnam draft. "It was sort of prison-like," Roberts recalls. "Their method of containing someone was to throw him in a locked room." The public-sector nurses started commenting that guitar strumming did not figure in his job description. Roberts got the hint and began looking around for work. A friend mentioned that nearby McLean, far better endowed than the struggling state hospital, actually had a music therapy department. But they did not have a sitar-playing cool guy; as it happened, McLean and Roberts had been looking for each other.

McLean had three practice rooms, each with its own piano, and was perfectly happy to turn the cafeteria over to any of the four bands that Roberts organized—the Zoo, the Strawberry Discharge, and Ronnie and the Waverley Squares (McLean overlooks Waverley Square)—and most famously, Sister Kate's Soul Stew and Submarine Sandwich Shoppe, headlined by Kate Taylor. The

Sandwich Shoppe played for money at Brandeis, at a Cambridge peace fair, and for a "social" at the Institute of Living, a mental hospital in Hartford, Connecticut. Roberts was not exactly sure what he was doing, but whatever he was doing, it was working. One catatonic patient, a gifted saxophone player, began communicating first with fellow band members and only later with his therapists. One of the bands became a long-running group therapy session, trying for its members but ultimately useful in resolving shared conflicts. Ronnie of the Waverley Squares was a Janis Joplin–like blues belter. "They couldn't give her enough Thorazine on the unit, but in music therapy, she was normal," Roberts remembers. Kate Taylor was revealed to be a hauntingly mellifluous singer, and she signed a recording contract soon after leaving the hospital.

"Some of the psychiatrists were hip to the fact that real therapy was taking place," says Roberts, who now pursues his singing career with his wife in Redbird, Colorado. "People were getting better, but I didn't know or care why it was working. I was just experimenting in the dark. These kids needed to express themselves through loud rock music, and it worked. I was putting in sixty, seventy, eighty hours a week. I was completely enthralled by what was going on." Roberts prepared a lengthy presentation on his band therapies for his academic mentor, who just happened to be Morris Schwartz of Brandeis, the same Morris Schwartz who coauthored *The Mental Hospital* with Alfred Stanton and the "Morrie" of *Tuesdays with Morrie*. Roberts's report included interviews with his performers, most of whom testified to finding extraordinary release with their bands. A vocalist named Laura told Roberts, "It's magic, almost. I mean, I have said that I'm going to kill myself in the morning, and then in the afternoon I'm singing my heart out. It's brought me time and time again out of depression." Understandably, some band members found the interpersonal dynamics overwhelming. When Roberts asked a keyboard player named Tom what it was like to perform in the band, Tom answered,

It's a drag, because you work for months and months and then you get into these hassles like who is loudest, who is soft. . . . I've always approached it as work. A lot of people think playing in a band is all fun and games but it isn't, it's work. It forces you to relate to other people, to consider how other people are feeling. It's very difficult to go ahead as though everything was a machine; you're working with people. For me the communication is with the music because I have difficulty in talking.

Before dropping out of Brandeis, Roberts's roommate had been an academically gifted history student named Jon Landau, who had musical ambitions of his own. Landau had his own band, and when Roberts came over to his house, the music therapist started talking up the talents of a severely withdrawn vocalist and guitar player, Livingston Taylor—James's and Kate's younger brother. Livingston was at the Arlington School and was supplementing his musical education at the Berklee School of Music in the Back Bay. The rest, as it were, is history. Landau forsook his own musical ambitions and produced his first record, *Livingston Taylor*, a beautiful collection of ballads that included at least one song with a McLean theme: "Doctor Man." A second Landau-Taylor collaboration, *Liv*, included "Carolina Day," with the words memorializing Livingston's therapist, Dr. Harvey Shein. Landau, who had been working as a rock critic at the *Boston Real Paper*, went on to become one of the most famous and powerful music producers of all time when he abandoned journalism to manage the career of a singer who, he believed, represented "the future of rock and roll": Bruce Springsteen.

∽

The Taylors were blessed—or cursed—with fame, but they were not the only successful musicians sojourning at McLean. As a Harvard undergraduate, Clay Jackson had played bluegrass guitar and mandolin with the Charles River Boys in the early 1960s and had backed up a crystal-voiced young folksinger named Joan Baez, who occasionally played concerts at the hospital. "She was a skinny little black-haired girl who had a voice you could hear for two blocks," says Jackson, whose life journey took him from Cambridge to London to Tangier to McLean and now back to his family home in Kerrville, Texas, where he is looking forward to receiving his first Social Security check: "I've sort of made an effort not to contribute to society," he says. The godson of James Taylor's father Isaac, John Sheldon, also ended up at McLean with Kate and Livingston, and after touring with James in the mid-1980s, he has carved out a successful performing career in western Massachusetts. After graduating from the Arlington School, Sheldon was approached by a young musician named Van Morrison to help him record a new album. "It was very odd," Sheldon remembers:

Van was living in Boston. "Brown-eyed Girl" was a hit, but Van didn't have any money because his record company—well, that's a whole other story. Anyway, he was broke. He had a band, but he didn't have a guitar player, because the guitar player had been murdered. I didn't know that at the time. That was just one of the strange things that surrounded Van.

I never did audition. I left my phone number with his manager, and he told me to check back with them. A little later I got call from this manager, asking me, "Where do you live?" I said, "Cambridge." "Can we come over?" I was seventeen years old, nobody had heard me play, I had been living in the hospital, so there was no one they could have talked to. . . .

So they come over to my parents' house—Van, the manager, and the bass player, and we went down to the basement, which is my band room, and we started playing music. I'd been playing the blues all winter, and Van loves the blues, so I got the job.

John is a superb guitarist whose recordings have something of the outlaw edge that David Bromberg brought to the early Bob

Dylan records. Now in his mid-forties, his mannerisms are those of the classic McLean graduate: He is jittery, funny, smart, and direct, and he is raising two children in the Pioneer Valley near Amherst. Thirty years ago, when he was just sixteen years old, he spent the summer touring New England with Morrison's band. Life with Van was never dull:

> Van tried to move into my house, but my Mom wouldn't let him. Then one day he shows up and says he's had a dream, and in the dream he's supposed to get rid of all the electric instruments. So the drummer gets fired because he's too loud, and we start rehearsing with bass and acoustic guitars. They start working on stuff like "Madame George," but I'm getting really bored, because I want to play rock and roll, I want to play loud.
>
> Then Warner Brothers signs him up, and it's time to go to New York and make a record. I'm seventeen and living at home—I really couldn't go with him. At that age, being in New York and depending on him . . . I just knew I couldn't depend on him.

Van Morrison's train left the station, and John Sheldon was not on it. The ethereal, acoustic album that Morrison cut for Warner Brothers turned out to be *Astral Weeks,* which some cognoscenti insist is one of the greatest rock records of all time. As it happened, McLean was represented on the album. The haunting flute solos that backstop songs like "Cyprus Avenue" and "Madame George" were provided by John Payne, a talented Harvard musician who interrupted his undergraduate studies to obtain a McLean "degree." As one doctor explained to me, with a knowing smile, "Music therapy at McLean was the path to greatness."

∞

Most of the young people who fetched up at McLean hailed from the social elite: Payne was a cousin of Robert Lowell; Isaac Taylor was a well-to-do doctor who worked for a time as dean of the medical school at the University of North Carolina. The son of John Marquand, at the time one of America's best-known novelists, was at McLean, as was the daughter of the legendary cartoonist Al Capp. Peppered elsewhere on the wards were Yankee Forbeses, a department store heiress, a Mafia don-in-waiting, and so on. "It was the great Cambridge sociology experiment," remarks Susanna Kaysen, author of the McLean memoir *Girl, Interrupted,* by which she means the warehousing of the troubled children of the well-to-do. Kaysen's own father was running Princeton's Institute for Advanced Study when she was hospitalized. "The old definition of the Proper Bostonian used to be someone who lived on Beacon Hill and had an uncle in McLean," Merton Kahne says. "As the clientele got younger, I used to joke that we were redefining the Proper Bostonian. Now it was someone at McLean who had an uncle on Beacon Hill."

The McLean youth movement was a response to what an economist might call a market opportunity. Psychiatry was a booming field, flush with confidence in its therapeutic powers. Doctors were pouring out of the medical schools and were looking for patients to analyze. Many insurance companies were paying for up to six months of inpatient care, and the field of adolescent psychiatry was burgeoning. And there was no shortage of troubled young people. The 1960s need no introduction here: Drugs, rebelliousness, and rejection of parental authority were the order of the day, especially in the socioeconomic strata that had access to psychiatric care. (In her official history of the hospital, Silvia Sutton remarks that "delinquent adolescents from less-advantaged homes had other destinies, such as reform school.") Conveniently, doctors developed a catchall diagnosis for their teenage clientele: "adolescent turmoil." "These were people who probably wouldn't be considered severe enough to be hospitalized now," says Dr. Michael Sperber, who worked on South Belknap and Bowditch during the 1960s. "Their curse was that somebody had some money in the family. It wasn't like managed care is today. There was a lot of money around, and as long as people had a bank account, you'd find something that they should work on."

Barbara Schwartz, a social worker who started at McLean in 1962, remembers that the young people began to invade the hospital in the early 1960s, at the end of the Stanton era, even before the well-documented scourges of drugs, sex, and rock and roll:

> The parents were in great distress. They had lost control. The kids were running away, doing all kinds of things. Now I shudder when I think of who was hospitalized. It was a difficult group because we didn't know what we were doing. I mean, we thought we did. If I only knew then what I know now, some of those kids would never have been admitted to that hospital, they would never have had to go through that kind of an experience. It saddens me. It was a shame.

Not surprisingly, there was no small amount of cynicism among the young people concerning the hospital's motivations. I interviewed a successful forty-something media executive in lower Manhattan who was still bristling with anger, both at his father for sending him to McLean and at the hospital for diagnosing him with an unspecified "character disorder." He showed me a photograph of himself in a football uniform and with long hair. "I was a hippie," he remembered.

> I hated jocks, and I didn't fit into any group. I hated most drugs—except for pot—but that didn't matter, because there wasn't any distinction between someone who used marijuana and someone who used heroin. As far as they were concerned, you were in the "drug culture." I refused to cut my hair, and I could have stopped smoking pot at any time. To have a hospital say I had a character disorder was a complete scam. McLean was scandalous to me. I don't think anyone ever spent the night there and didn't get diagnosed with a character disorder.

When she retrieved her McLean file to write *Girl, Interrupted,* Susanna Kaysen noticed that her diagnosis was "borderline personality disorder" (BPD), another controversial catchall, popularized and promoted by McLean's own John Gunderson, the same doctor who managed the decade-long schizophrenia study for Alfred Stanton in the 1960s.* To this day, Kaysen, like many members of the psychiatric profession, is not exactly sure what her diagnosis meant: "BPD—a psychiatrist once told me that's what they call people whose lifestyles they don't like." John Sheldon also managed to see his case file. "If you look at my notes, it just said 'adolescent turmoil.' It's not even clearly diagnosed. The thinking was, 'This guy's having a tough adolescence. Let's lock him up so he doesn't hurt himself.'"

The McLean party line, articulated to me in an interview by Shervert Frazier, the cerebral Texas doctor who ascended to the post of psychiatrist-in-chief in 1972, was that the kids were on drugs. Sitting in Frazier's well-appointed office, decorated with an old-fashioned painting of a sailing ship on the wall, I could not help feeling that I was talking to one of my own parents or to one of any of my generation's parents, indeed, of every generation's parents: well-meaning, avuncular, out of touch. At age seventy-nine, Frazier has kept himself in marvelous shape; he swims and lifts weights, and I first met him hiking the antique, oak-paneled corridors of the administration building during the ten-minute breaks between his therapeutic appointments. His speech, for all its fineries of thought, still twangs of the Lone Star State. He speaks in clear paragraphs; indeed, when he later lost his job in a plagiarism scandal, his defenders suggested that his habit of dictating finished journal copy probably did him in, so adept was he at assimilating materials that he had read or heard, that his brain

---

*BPD has occasioned a good deal of skepticism even within the psychiatric profession. The 1999 *Dictionary of Psychology* calls BPD a "vague phrase for a group of psychological conditions that are characterized between normality and neurosis, between neurosis and psychosis, or between normal intelligence and mental retardation." In his 1998 *History of Psychiatry*, Dr. Edward Shorter mocks BPD as "Woody Allen syndrome." The diagnosis does crop up at the strangest times. For instance, in her 1999 bestseller *Diana: In Search of Herself*, journalist Sally Bedell Smith cites "compelling evidence" that the late Princess Diana had a borderline personality disorder.

never processed their provenance. So here is Frazier, McLean's psychiatrist-in-chief for twelve years, on the subject of his rambunctious, youthful charges:

> These young people were usually from well to do families who wanted another opinion about what was going on with their children. Mainly, the families didn't know how many drugs or what drugs they were using; they just knew there had been a noticeable change in personality, and they wanted to know what caused the change in personality and what could we do about it.
>
> As you know, street drugs were readily available and were cheap at that time, and people were going to India and to ashrams, people were joining politically inspired groups and cults, too. Essentially we had a lot of adolescents around here with forty, sometimes four hundred LSD trips, and a lot of brain damage as a result. We saw use of every kind of drug under the sun—angel dust, LSD, Ecstasy, drugs that been around for years and years and years—plus all the street drugs including marijuana, hashish, cocaine, heroin, which they called "H." These people were addicted and their behavior while under the influence of drugs was erratic. They were not themselves, and at times they were dangerous to themselves and to others. Their friends didn't recognize them and vice versa. Many of them had disowned their families. Nobody in the old-line families had ever seen anything like it—all they ever did was drink martinis.

One of Frazier's contemporaries, Dr. Alan Stone, weighed in along similar lines in a lengthy review of the movie *Girl, Interrupted* made from Kaysen's book. Stone was a resident at McLean and later became director of residency training there before defecting to Harvard Law School, where he now teaches. He writes of the 1960s kids:

> These were kids who dropped acid every day and found their own reality; some also did heroin, speed, and barbiturates (cocaine had not yet arrived). Some actually had psychiatric disorders, which they were

treating with their own drugs in their own ways. Feeling anxious or lonely—smoke pot. Worried that you're losing your mind—take acid and see how far you can go. But most troubling to their parents were the self-destructive behaviors, not just having casual sex with strangers but burning themselves with cigarettes, cutting their arms with razors, making their own primitive tattoos, and worse. One psychiatric pundit said that "hippiephrenia" was replacing schizophrenia.

They looked and acted crazy by conventional standards but they did not fit into any of our diagnostic categories. We eventually had to create a new diagnosis for patients like Kaysen: Borderline Personality Disorder. It was by no means easy for us to decide when someone had crossed the border from hippie to hippiephrenia.

The records of the time are full of the kind of well-intentioned floundering that has always characterized the older generation's attempts to understand their children. One former administrator gave me a copy of a 1968 panel presentation entitled "An Adolescent Program Needed." It amounts to fifty pages of hand-wringing on the part of top doctors and the teachers at the Arlington School about the obvious successes the boys and girls were enjoying in their ongoing battles with authority. The all-important therapy sessions were used as excuses for blowing off classes and exams, and students lied to their doctors about their school commitments. During the panel discussion, the director of the Arlington School laments that four students wangled a half-day pass into Cambridge to see the Beatles movie *Yellow Submarine* by informing their ward administrator that school ended at noon that day. In fact, an important chemistry exam had been scheduled. During the same year, administrators convened a "Youth Forum," summoning adolescent patients to the coffee shop to vent their concerns about life in the hospital. The meetings, which were held weekly for several months, were predictably chaotic. The young people wanted "more freedom" but had no idea how to get it. The doctors encouraged them to take various initiatives, but this was, after all, a mental hospital, not a Marine Corps barracks. The most vociferous complainers rarely attended two meetings in a row; invitations to certain doctors were never written; the patients bemoaned their sense of helplessness. When the administrators fretted that the young patients did not participate in hospital outings, they heard the obvious feedback: We don't want to go to Crane's Beach or to the Museum of Fine Arts or to Fenway Park. "The trouble with hospital trips is that they aren't of interest to the younger people," one patient said. "I bet if you had a trip to the Jimi Hendrix concert, you'd have fifty or sixty patients showing up."

It is easy sport, poking fun at overcredentialed authority figures who have to coin nonsense words like "hippiephrenia" to describe young people's psychological disturbances. But if doctors like Frazier and Stone wax pompous and uninformed about the children of the 1960s, then where does the truth lie? Certainly a huge percentage of the hospitalized youngsters experimented with some drugs; they were hardly alone. But only a tiny fraction of young people ended up in mental hospitals. So if drugs did not cause mental disturbances, what did? Or if heavy drug use testified to some deeper anxiety, what was it? Peter Storkerson, a man now in his late forties who spent eight months in McLean in 1967, thought the problems began when the younger generation failed to live up to the expectations of what is now portentously called the Greatest Generation. His own father played football in college with the legendary Knute Rockne and ran a successful high-tech business that employed 1,500 people. Six feet tall, Peter is thin-boned and slight. "My father was the model I was given, one I had no way of fulfilling. In my family, you grew up with a certain set of expectations about how you are going to perform, how you are going to succeed, and if it doesn't happen to be appropriate, you have no real alternatives." Barbara Schwartz was Susanna Kaysen's social worker, and she remembers the family's disenchantment with their daughter's life choices: "Her father had wanted her hospitalized because she was a stubborn child. She didn't want to go to college. That was anathema to him. He couldn't tolerate that.

After all, he was at the Institute for Advanced Studies at Princeton. So there must be something wrong with her head for her not to want to go to college." A man whose first three names are Pierrepont Edward Stuyvesant used words like Storkerson's to describe the anguish felt by the children of the aristocracy, many of whom landed in McLean. This man's father had never worked, inhabited a huge seaside manor, and confiscated Roosevelt dimes from his son, so much did he hate the "socialist" depredations of the New Deal. "The sons and daughters of the old families couldn't commiserate with anyone," Pierrepont told me. "They had their own confusions and incoherence but the parents wouldn't speak to them about it. There was this terrific need to talk about it."

If the kids were not sick in the conventional sense, then one has to ask: How were they treated, and more important, how could they show evidence of being "cured" and get out? The treatment had not changed much over the years, although of course the young people were not subjected to Scotch douches, insulin therapy, or electroshock. Many of them were still medicated with Thorazine, the powerful antipsychotic drug left over from the 1950s. The drug effectively sedated even the most hyperactive teenager and generated bizarre side effects, such as the aimless "Thorazine shuffle," an occasionally lolling tongue, and the "Thorazine tan." (The drug heightens the skin's sensitivity to the sun, so on their occasional outings to the beach or the New Hampshire woods, the boys and girls had to be extra careful to wear long-sleeve shirts and pants to avoid quickly baking to a golden ochre.) "It's really a heavy and stultifying tranquilizer," James Taylor recalls. "It's a blunt instrument, and a very heavy-handed way of dealing with mental health problems. It felt like someone had cast my head in concrete."

But the primary course of therapy remained the hour or hours of talk psychotherapy, and milieu therapy, referring to the generally supportive caregivers, the gorgeous grounds, and the absence of siblings and parents, who were sometimes assigned the fashionable term "schizophrenogenic." Of course, milieu therapy cut both ways. Many socially maladapted troublemakers suddenly found themselves in the company of other troublemakers, and antisocial behavior was reinforced. In some respects, life on the inside was not so different from life on the outside. As in every college dorm, the KLH stereo was the centerpiece furnishing for each room, and drugs–the supposed root of all psychological evil–were available. Rob Perkins remembers blasting the Chambers' Brothers raucous anthem "Time Has Come Today" ("Time has come today / Young hearts can go their way. . . . / I don't care what others say / They say we don't listen anyway") at top volume with friends of his inside a locked room on Bowditch until aides came and broke the door down. The perpetrators would lose their stereos, their albums, and all privileges. One after another, they regained their possessions and their freedoms–and then pulled the same stunt all over again.

Some of the Arlington School students were outpatients and went home at night and brought dope back into the hospital; some of the ward aides shared their stashes. Subjected to frequent checks, the patients evolved ever more inventive hiding places: a toothpaste tube; a hole in a windowsill; under the pin of the ninth golf hole, which sat smack in front of the administration building. "There was this real country club aspect to the whole place," John Sheldon told me.

> You could hide anything, you could get anything, somebody was always going into town and coming back with something. McLean was the first place I ever got marijuana. The first night I was there, I was in the bathroom and this guy came in and said, "How cool are you?" I said, "What are you talking about?" And he said, "You want to get stoned?" So that's when I started smoking pot! Isn't it a riot? I don't know whether to laugh or cry, when I think about it.

Once someone was in, the key question became how to get out. In theory, one could just walk out, the way James Taylor did. But with no money and no support system, there was nowhere to go. Most families would accept their children back into the fold only after they had been "cured" by McLean, that is, formally discharged into a halfway house or back to their homes. Peter Storkerson got out because after six months he still had not been assigned a psychotherapist. "I told them 'This is my money, I'm here voluntarily, you haven't done anything for me, I'm gone.'" For John Sheldon, it took somewhat longer to arrive at a similar realization:

They're not going to let you out of there until you do what they want. You know you're not crazy but you have to figure out what they want. . . . First of all, you figure out that your parents aren't going to come get you, and then you get really angry, because you're left there with these lunatics. You're just really, really pissed—and that's why they don't let you out! So you start finding other people who are pissed, and hang around with them. You look for people who are intelligent, who are rebellious and pissed off, who at least have a sense of humor. . . . a lot of them are substance-abuse people, like alcoholics, because they're all smarter, believe it or not, and they're funnier, they're more intelligent. I think they're so smart and they see through things so clearly that they have to take something to blot it out.

I hung out with those people, but that doesn't help you get out.

After a year, I finally figured it out. I put on the act to get out, and it worked! It was just what you'd expect, it was the simplest thing in the world. You say you're really thinking about your future, and that you're really going to work hard in school, and you're really excited about the opportunities out there in the world . . . all that stuff. . . . And you sit differently, and you talk differently. You stop slouching in the chair, you sit up straight; it's like Oliver North in front of the discharge panel.

It was all quite simple, in the end. Figure out what society deems to be sane behavior and copy it. You act like you are getting better, and you will get better. And eventually you will grow up.

Diagnosis: "Hippiephrenia"

⌘

When I began researching this book, I befriended "June Tavistock," a woman my age who had spent some time at McLean. June was just fifteen years old when she arrived at McLean with the conventional diagnosis—"adjustment reaction of adolescence"—stamped on the front jacket of her case record folder. In the fall of 1966, when she was sent to Belmont, June was plenty mixed up. An urban girl from a prominent, liberal Chicago family, she was predictably shocked by the death of her gregarious, popular father. Her mother's subsequent remarriage forced the family to relocate, parachuting June into unfamiliar schools, first in the United States and then abroad. Despite an above-average IQ, June was not thriving in school. A psychiatrist friend of the family suggested McLean.

June is okay now. After McLean, she graduated from college, launched a successful career, and has published two books. She is smart, she is funny, and she can be plenty discombobulated. I was once talking with her on a cell phone when she blurted out, "Oh my God, I'm driving down a one-way street!" I later learned that she passed her Massachusetts driving test while living at McLean.

Like many former patients, June asked McLean for a copy of her case record and agreed to let me read and quote from it, with a few identifying details changed. It provides a fascinating keyhole through which to observe life on the wards during the late 1960s.

McLean Hospital and June Tavistock first made each other's acquaintance just before noon on the morning of November 10, 1966. For the next eighteen months, the nurses in Codman Hall entered notes on her behavior three times a day. Here is the first of them:

Admitted to COD1 at 11:45 AM—fifteen year old 5′ 5″ 105lb female with brown hair & blue eyes—dressed nicely—very talkative & cooperative to admission procedure—apparently knows all about mental hospital set-ups through friends & books she's read—Visited w mother in PM—appears quite intelligent & probably will try to control us & will pick up any flaw in the system e.g., why can we have glass such as vases, shampoo bottles out & yet you [nurses] have to keep eyebrow tweezers—Also commented that "Don't you believe if someone has a strong intent to commit suicide they'll do it no matter what protection anyone gives?—I do—it's a good thing I love myself."

McLean was still doing forty-day work-ups, meaning that the doctors spent five to six weeks of interviewing and testing just to diagnose new patients. By mid-December, two psychiatrists signed off on her eighteen-page case report, based on interviews with June, her mother, her brother, and several psychiatrists who had treated June during the previous twelve years. The result was a minibiography of a fifteen-year-old girl. The examining doctors surmised [correctly, I think] that the chronic illnesses and death of June's father, a wealthy department store magnate and popular philanthropist, had traumatized the young girl and her immediate family. The doctors made note of the "comfortable trust fund" underwriting June's hospital stay and mentioned the largesse of her uncle Rudolph, the fund's trustee. They confirmed the "adjustment reaction" diagnosis and laid out a plan for treatment: "First and foremost, we intend to support patient's wish to remain at McLean Hospital." June had already entered the Arlington School and the doctors wanted her to continue. For therapy, they prescribed the mild tranquilizer Librium and intended for June to see a staff psychiatrist several times a week.

Prognosis: If we can lure June into participation in a relatively stable home environment on one of the Halls at McLean, it would seem that, over a period of time, she would gain immeasurably by this living experience. Particularly important, would seem to be that we must show a concern for her. This would include letting her know that we would be willing to take care of her even if she shows regressive and disturbed behavior which she would set up in order to get transferred to [the female disturbed ward] East House, or even if she does not act like a buffoonery [sic] which she seems to need to do, according to her, in order to get the immediate, proper attention that she craves. . . . Therefore, assuming we can offer her the milieu and controls which she so desperately needs and craves, the prognosis should be quite good. However, the length of time which we will have for this job will be determining.

The subsequent nurses' notes are mercilessly thorough. No appointment, no friendship, no spat, no mood swing, no reading material ("Reading a book on 'This Is Mental Illness' w vivid case histories and therapy") nor sortie outside the hospital ("Admitted movie [*Who's Afraid of Virginia Woolf*] had depressed her") would go unnoted in the narrow-lined nurses' register. Viewed from the outside, June's life does not seem half bad; she takes cabs to visit friends in the Boston area, she flies to New York and Chicago for vacations, she cooks up a storm in the Codman kitchen and occasionally jawbones the nurses into taking care of her cat, Ripple—although the hospital pharmacy draws the line at filling veterinary prescriptions. Late in her stay, the nurses catch June and two equally underage friends sharing a bottle of champagne in the Codman conference room.

But of course this is a mental hospital, not a summer camp. Conflicts with nurses, with doctors, and sometimes with other young patients frequently flare up:

12/18/66: Very hostile. Wrote letter to Dr. Ross requesting Dr. Z. as administrator as Dr. H. doesn't understand her. Says if she doesn't get what she wants she'll put in a three-day notice. Very hostile—much noise, objected to 1/2 hour checks saying that she didn't need to be checked, she wasn't cutting her wrists under the covers. Piled covers against door in shape of body. When told that if she didn't conform to expectations of behavior of COD patients, she would have to go elsewhere, she quieted down.

12/22/66: Told of room change by charge nurse. Reaction was violent to say the least. Turned in a 3-day notice @ 4:27 because of staff conspiracy to ruin her. Screamed at any & all staff members who approached. In the midst of this mother placed a timely call to say she'd arrived in town. Told by staff if she didn't settle down she'd have to go to East House & she was setting up a situation in which only she lost—saw Dr. H—3-day notice retracted at 6:15—doctor on call and superintendent notified both times—plus room change was not made. Patient pulled herself together miraculously & out to dinner w mother.

At times, the nurses make note of June's "loud and un-ladylike" behavior; but as the months progress, the tantrums diminish and June's friendships on the ward strengthen and develop:

4/4/67: Being just an angel—quiet and sweet. Was very pleased that Sarah asked her to talk w her in eve—Said she "felt like being good." Strongly complimented—appreciated that nurse knew that she felt useful + needed + that was reason for "good." Very funny lying on floor trying to "quietly" scare new aide but couldn't stop giggling. To bed @ end of TV movie.

During a brief stay at the Massachusetts General Hospital, moved by the concern of her psychiatrist, nurses, and fellow patients who had come to visit her, June said, "she loves McLean and never ever wants to leave." Three months later, June took a week-long trip to Chicago and called in to the ward several times to catch up on gossip or just to check in: "4/16/67 called in 7 PM to say she misses everyone." Upon her return, "4/25/67 was met at the airport by staff member. Arrived on the hall. Was very happy to be back at McLean."

A certain cynicism attends any hospital's long-term treatment of wealthy patients who pay their bills in full and who subsidize the care of less fortunate souls. But in June's case, McLean worked to cut the umbilical cord that was tethering the young patient to the hospital. June overnighted outside the hospital with several sets of foster parents, never very satisfactorily. Some conflict or another always seemed to develop. For a time, June attended a progressive school that—this was 1968—was transforming itself into a commune. Her social worker and her mother reacted with horror:

> June has already spent several weekends and longer on trips sponsored by the school with various combinations of teachers, parents and students. During one such excursion to Washington, the group camped in Mrs. Tavistock's elegant apartment, and, according to Mrs. Tavistock, were an unkempt, hippie-looking aggregation of dirty people who never took a shower the whole time they were there.
>
> June explained that part of the philosophy of Tord and his group includes the idea that human odors are good odors. . . .

But the fact was, June had graduated from McLean. Her discharge summary served as her transcript:

> Her behavior on the hall throughout her hospitalization improved markedly as a result of therapy and milieu. Although still alert, aggressive and in effect "the life of the hall" she has been much more able to contain her hostile and aggressive outbursts which were so characteristic when she would become frustrated or frightened. . . . She is now able to express her concerns over entering womanhood and to ask relevant questions concerning how one relates to the opposite sex. She has been increasingly able to accept the advice and criticism of her peers in relation to her impulsive and sometimes inappropriate behavior concerning her relations with men. On discharge the patient continues to be fully oriented showing no evidence of delusional or hallucinatory experiences.

∞

The teenagers who invaded McLean in the late 1960s and early 1970s changed the character of the hospital forever. They blasted their music in the halls, they took dope, and they engineered frequent escapes, which almost always resulted in a slump-shouldered taxicab ride back to the hospital from either Waverley or Harvard Square. The musician Clay Jackson told me he felt an obligation to escape "because everybody did that, and I'm a traditionalist at heart. . . . I got a bottle and took off for New York. I rented a hotel room in Times Square and looked at the weirdoes for a couple of days. Then I took a return bus and arrived back at the hospital just as they were about to call out the state police." Jeff Garland of Cape Elizabeth, Maine, committed by his parents at age fifteen, escaped from McLean eight times, unsuccessfully. Private investigators sent by his parents inevitably returned him to Belmont. The ninth time was the charm. With $150 borrowed from wealthy friends on Bowditch, he first hid with two ex-patients in the Boston suburb of Brookline and then hitched up with another ex-patient in New York City. From there he moved to Minnesota. "Who would think of looking in Minnesota?" asks Garland, who is now a community activist in Hawaii. "Nobody's crazy enough to go out there—only somebody who had escaped from McLean Hospital."

At the tender age of twenty-two, a gorgeous, demure blonde named Maria Pugatch was the head nurse on Bowditch, the hall for male disturbed patients. Not infrequently her teenage charges, sporting their trademark uniform of black jeans, bare chests, and thick leather belts (when permitted) informed her they intended to "riot" and warned her to seek shelter. She did nothing of the sort and staved off many a putative disturbance by squaring her hands against her hips and daring the boys to act out. Male patients had no qualms about assaulting male aides and nurses, but they hardly ever harmed a woman.

Some floors of South Belknap—*Girl, Interrupted* is set on the second floor—and East House, where the female disturbed patients lived, were far wilder than the boys' dorms. One favorite Belknap trick was to yank the fire alarms, which brought a pack of Belmont firemen onto the ward. There a clutch of girls would be waiting for them, hanging from the exposed ceiling pipes, wearing no underwear. One patient, a woman who was caring for her newborn baby on South Belknap, remembered one of the venerable McLean dowagers, Agnes Sweeney:

> This woman was just as imperious as they come, she was in her seventies, and she was not to be trifled with. I often wondered what Agnes thought when all these kids came, because they were terrifying, they were loud, they were obscene, they were saying words that most of us had not ever heard spoken out loud. Those five girls were just holy terrors! These were scary kids, they were rambunctious and loud, running up and down and screaming at the nurses, unhappy and scared.

And of course the kids were doing kid things: smoking dope, sneaking out to the woods for furtive sexual encounters (probably more talked about than consummated), and using "privileges" to get into Harvard Square or Boston and touch base with 1960s culture. A black nurse on Belknap took Kate Taylor and two friends to an Otis Redding concert and to the Roxbury nightclub Estelle's after the show. "We sat there, these three white gals and our watcher from Roxbury," Kate recalls. Another popular destination was the Boston Tea Party, a concert venue for A-list acts from all over the country. Rob Perkins remembers one outing to see the Jeff Beck group at the Tea Party when he and a group of friends helped push their friend Kim, a famous Bowditch escape artist, through a bathroom window. (He was later caught.) Munson Hicks, who was performing with the Cambridge improvisational troupe The Proposition and also teaching at the Arlington School, remembers appearing in a New Year's Eve bill at the Tea Party with the Grateful Dead and his pupil Livingston Taylor: "There we were in coats and ties during the day, and backstage with the Dead at night!"

Dr. Michael "Mickey" Robinson, who ran Bowditch, occasionally treated his disturbed charges to a week at a summer camp in New Hampshire or to a skiing expedition in the winter. Bowditch—"no country club," several of my informants agreed—was for hard cases: heavily medicated, occasionally violent male patients. And yet, to the astonishment of the McLean higher-ups, the trips generally came off without a hitch. Robinson insisted that the boys "earn" their trips by holding car washes or performing chores, so they would see the connection between work and leisure. (In reality, their parents paid for most of the travel.) Participants remember the week at camp—to the extent that they remember it at all—as bucolic and restorative. Horseback riding, a classic McLean therapy when the stables were still active, intrigued the young men and supposedly schooled them in issues of power and control. "Horses were wonderful for these guys," says Maria Pugatch, who remembers handing out meds on horseback. "It was a good way to overcome your feeling of being frightened and to overcome your power feeling. The frightened ones would learn that the horse would do what you told it, and the ones who were into control would learn that there was no reason to hurt the horse." A few aides bunked down with the patients and doled out Thorazine caplets, washed down with Kool-Aid at night. Munson Hicks, now a successful actor, worked as an aide on Bowditch and described one of the ski trips to Waterville Valley for me. He remembered one of the patients becoming agitated when forced to wait in a long ski lift line. Munson paused for a moment, and we stared into each other's eyes. Pissed off at long ski lines? There's nothing mad about that!

The point of the trips, aside from pure recreation, was to see how the patients reacted to experiences in the "real world"—although the McLean patient's real world could be quite removed from everyday reality. Maria Pugatch occasionally donned her best dress and high heels and hopped in a hired car with a group of male patients headed for the Ritz to celebrate a birthday. A boy's parents would make the reservation, and Pugatch and her charges walked into the dining room like anyone else. Except for the individually labeled medication bottles in her purse, they could have been a well-to-do family out for a tasty meal.

There were many occasions where you'd be with someone who'd been walking around the ward pulling out pieces of his hair and mumbling nonsense, and they would walk into the Ritz and you wouldn't be able to tell. They had impeccable manners. The Ritz was of course a place they might have frequented. They were extremely wealthy, and they were used to this. The waiter would come around, and the patients would say, "Maria, what would you like?"

Occasionally you'd see somebody start to go off a little. A little mumbling, maybe rolling their eyes, or showing a tic or something. Then I would just pull out their medicine, each in a separate labeled bottle, and they would go to the men's room to take a pill.

There wasn't ever a time when these men didn't say, "I can't thank you enough for your discretion." Then they would be so sad, it was so gut-wrenching, because some of them of them would say, "I would really like to be here on a date with a young woman," and then they'd have to go back to McLean, and leave me at the ward door with a little nod.

Many former patients, the ones who got out of McLean in one piece, have positive memories of their times. "You had some of the most spirited people of our day in there—it was much more interesting than a lot of the progressive colleges of our time," said my media executive friend in New York City. After leaving McLean, talk-show host Ellen Ratner attended Goddard College and received a master's degree from Harvard. "I got more of an education at McLean than at Goddard, Harvard and covering the White House," she told me.

It was Nirvana for me. I was on a hall with all the Seven Sisters represented. I was in high Boston culture. Al Capp's daughter was there, Robert Lowell was there. I could go out any time I wanted, I had more freedom than any teenager I knew.

McLean Hospital seemed like a great option for me. And it was. It was one of the best experiences of my life.

Physician, Heal Thyself

"Did you hear about Dr. Shein?" they asked.

*In 1967, Walter Jackson Freeman, the father of the ice-pick lobot-*omy, published a book called *Psychiatrist: Personalities and Patterns.*
It is a generally undistinguished overview of the profession, for
the most part a collection of poorly written profiles of Freeman's
heroes, the biologically oriented therapists like Manfred Sakel,
the inventor of the insulin shock treatment, and António Egasmoniz, the Nobel Prize–winning lobotomy pioneer. Freeman, the
archetypal hands-on kind of guy, lumped Sigmund Freud, Otto
Rank, and Harry Stack Sullivan into one brief chapter called "The
Great Theorists." And yet, in a ghoulish final chapter entitled
"Mortido: The Death Instinct," Freeman hit on something. Eight
of Freud's closest disciples had killed themselves; why? He went
on to suggest that "suicide might be called a vocational hazard for
the psychiatrist."

Freeman was a crackpot enthusiast; maybe he was even a little mad.* But the mad often have special insights, and Freeman pursued this one as far as it would go. There was no literature on psychiatric suicide, so Freeman did his own research. He combed the obituary notices of the *Journal of the American Medical Association (JAMA)* to prove his point. When a reported cause of death seemed suspicious, he addressed the relevant state Bureau of Vital Statistics, with mixed results. Although his findings were far from scientific, they were provocative. He reported that 203 American psychiatrists had committed suicide in the seventy years from 1895 to 1965. He deduced, convincingly, that suicides were underreported by the medical profession and also that this seemed like a high number. As with his hurry-up-time's-a-wasting lobotomies in his medical office, his methodology was suspect. But yet again, his work commanded attention.

Perhaps understandably, there is very little literature on the subject of psychiatric suicide. In 1980, two California psychiatrists revisited Freeman's thesis, and—unlike most of his theories—it held up perfectly. Writing in the *Journal of Clinical Psychiatry,* Charles Rich and Ferris Pitts reported that "psychiatrists suicide regularly, year-by-year, at rates about twice those expected." They used American Medical Association records instead of the *JAMA* obituaries that Freeman combed through; the *JAMA* understated suicide rates by about 20 percent, according to Rich and Pitts. But even this report was misleading, because they were comparing psychiatrists' suicide rates to *doctors'* suicide rates, which are considerably higher than those for the general population. The two authors even allowed themselves a moment of what must have been unintentional levity: "The occurrence of suicides by psychia-

---

*At some length, Freeman dwelt on his hunch that Alfred Stanton's intellectual mentor, Harry Stack Sullivan, committed suicide in Paris in 1949. Freeman noted that Sullivan once predicted that he would die at the age of fifty-seven years, five months, and three days. Sullivan actually died at age fifty-six, but Freeman pointed out that if one counts Sullivan's "time of quickening"—in utero—then his prediction was accurate.

trists is quite constant year-to-year, indicating a relatively stable over-supply of depressed psychiatrists from which the suicides are produced."

Why do psychiatrists kill themselves? Many admit that they entered the profession to wrestle with their own demons—"to find out what was wrong with me," is the phrase I heard over and over again. Rich and Pitts confirmed this. Massaging their data, they hypothesized that one in every three psychiatrists suffered from a mood disorder like mania or depression. This, they wrote, is three times the incidence in the general population: "This would logically imply that psychiatry is depressing to the practitioner and/or physicians with affective disorder tend to select psychiatry as a specialty. For a variety of reasons, we believe the latter to be the case."

Mental illness can be infectious. Nurses, psychiatric aides, and therapists are hardly indifferent to their surroundings in the mental hospital, and many of them break down themselves. As the doctors are fond of saying: No one is immune.

∞

It is not uncommon for psychiatrists to check themselves into a sanitarium or hospital, although they usually seek shelter outside their practice area to avoid the possible embarrassment of meeting patients or students inside the hospital. Boston doctors might travel to the Yale–New Haven Hospital or to the bucolic surroundings of Austen Riggs in Stockbridge, in the heart of the Berkshire mountains.

But some ended up at McLean. One well-known patient was Dr. Doris Menzer-Benaron, a prominent member of the Boston Psychoanalytic Institute, who spent a good deal of time with the "crazy ladies" of Codman Hall. Benaron was married to a prominent local psychiatrist, and she had trained some of the doctors at

McLean. For understandable reasons, she was regarded with great empathy by doctors and patients alike.

Another sad case was that of Julia Altschule, who was married to Dr. Mark Altschule, a cardiologist who also functioned as McLean's one-man research laboratory from 1947 through the early 1960s. Julia had been a ballerina and assumed a curious Asian affect as she grew old at McLean, diagnosed as a chronic schizophrenic. She often wreathed herself in a black shawl, and wandered the grounds along "Julia's path," which took her from Codman Hall, behind Eliot Chapel, down over the Bowl, down to the Pleasant Street Lodge and back again. Julia would occasionally stop and talk with small children, as she did with Harold Williams's two-year-old son. What did they talk about? "God only knows," Williams now says. "I never heard a sane word come out of her."

Nurse Maria Pugatch remembers seeing Julia at the head of the grand staircase in Upham Hall, where she lived for a time: "Imagine how spooky it was to come into this building, and there at the top of the stairs is this short little woman dressed entirely in black, speaking in a kind of a tongue. Sometimes when you drove into the hospital, she would be standing on the top of a hill, casting spells on you. Everyone said she was a witch."

Huddled in a tiny, one-room lab in a tunnel just beneath the main administration building, her husband devoted much of his life to discovering a cure for his wife's illness. Working with pots and pans instead of test tubes and petri dishes, Altschule kept searching for the biological roots of his wife's illness. He experimented with different megavitamin recipes, occasionally tube-feeding them to catatonic schizophrenics in the hopes of mobilizing them. He also tried to isolate an extract of the pineal gland, which he injected into schizophrenics, hoping for a cure. "Like all therapy in schizophrenia, it worked in the beginning, or seemed to, and didn't lead anywhere," remembers Dr. Alfred Pope, a friend and colleague of Altschule's. "The pineal had been considered a vestigial organ that did nothing," Pope adds, "and Mark deserved credit for putting it on the map. It turned out to be a minute but important organ, especially in relation to sleep mechanisms." But it does not play a role in the neurobiology of schizophrenia.*

Worse tragedies than a doctor's wife's madness were to befall the hospital. On Father's Day, 1962, Williams, the hospital's doctor on call, decided to look in on a young resident named Wellington Cu, whom Williams himself had urged to transfer to McLean from a post in New York City. Cu had been depressed and acting strangely. He had broken up with his girlfriend and was also having problems with the immigration authorities, who had threatened to deport him back to the Philippines. Cu, an ethnic Chinese, had been raised by his grandmother in Shanghai and did not speak Tagalog. As it happened, McLean's suicide epidemic was in full swing. Cu's friend and fellow resident Dr. John Ellenberg thinks as many as eight patients had killed themselves during the previous year. "There was this business of suicides going around," he says, "and we were trying to figure out among ourselves why this was happening." Dr. Captane Thomson encouraged Cu to emigrate to Canada, and the two men even bought a footlocker together. "'That will be my casket,' is what he said," Thomson remembers. "He was dropping broad hints. We said, 'Come on Wellington, don't be so discouraged. We know you can get through this.' You know how you try to jolly people along and help them out. None of us thought he would take his own life."

Mounting the stairs of Waverley House, the white clapboard three-story colonial home where the cheery young assistant Earl Bond had lived in 1909, Williams had a premonition of fear. "I had the feeling that someone was dead there," says Williams, "and there he was lying on the bed." On Father's Day, Cu had taken his

---

*Altschule left McLean under a cloud, suggesting in a videotaped interview that he was persona non grata on the psychoanalytically oriented campus. While there, he made one discovery of lasting importance. As the hospital's director of internal medicine, he was alarmed by the number of patient deaths during electroshock therapy. He correctly deduced that an injection of the depressant atropine might relax the cardiovascular system before shock; atropine is still used for this purpose.

own life with an overdose of barbiturates—intended to be passed on to Cu's sister—that his father had mailed to him from the Philippines. In a suicide note, Cu thanked all of his friends and wrote that if it hadn't been for them he would have killed himself sooner. Then he explained that he had ingested twenty-six Seconal tablets, "one for every miserable year of my life." Ellenberg remembers that the note carefully did not blame "this person or that person, so it was a list of everybody who could have possibly intervened. He accused everybody he could by saying he didn't blame them."

In the presence of the dead body, Williams recalls, the two doctors had no idea what to do. "Luckily, Ellenberg had some religious training, and he had that to fall back on. We went back downstairs, he put on his hat and said, 'Let's have something to eat and say a prayer.'" In a neighboring bedroom, Ellenberg sang kaddish for the deceased Chinese-Filipino resident. "Then," says Williams, "we wondered whom we should call first. We decided to call Stanton and ruin his entire month." Once at the scene, even Stanton was not quite clear about the proper procedure for disposing of a corpse. Eventually they located an Episcopal priest who knew how to handle these things.

"Wellington once said to me that the worst thing you can do to someone is to kill yourself on his doorstep," Williams recalls. "Well, that's exactly what he did to McLean." More than a decade later, another doctor took aim at the hospital and hit squarely on the mark.

∽

During the years that I interviewed people for this book, I joked that I was actually building an impressive archive of tape-recorded restaurant and coffee shop sounds, what radio reporters call actuality. And indeed, I have put together a sort of audio field guide to clattering spoons, crashing crockery, and the repeat visits from solicitous serving people, asking me and my interviewee if everything was all right. My interview with Dr. Stephen Bergman falls into this category, a "sounds of Starbucks" classic. We met in a mini-mall near our homes in Newton, Massachusetts, a city that boasts the largest per capita infestation of psychiatrists and psychologists in America. Newton, inevitably dubbed a "leafy suburb" when sports announcers come by to cover a Boston College football game, is quite precious. Indeed, there was a protest of sorts when Starbucks opened the location where Bergman and I decided to meet, as the Seattle-based giant was invading the territory of a popular, previously existing coffee bar around the corner.

Bergman, a tall, imposing, bald eagle of a man, is in his mid-fifties and has written three novels under the pen name Samuel Shem. He is well known in the Boston medical establishment, if not well liked. His first novel, *House of God,* was a bawdy, artfully written roman à clef about his year spent training in the emergency room of Boston's Beth Israel Hospital. Relentlessly realistic (and thus unflattering) in its portrayal of the medical establishment, it alienated virtually every important doctor in the city, sold well, and has since become a classic among medical students. Bergman's third novel was *Mount Misery,* a similarly disguised account of his psychiatric residency at McLean, where he developed an instant attachment to an intense, cigar-smoking young administrator named Harvey Shein.

Bergman picks up his story after his stint at Beth Israel:

I was all set to go Mass Mental [Massachusetts Mental Health Center] for my psychiatric training. But I thought okay, I'll take a look at McLean. Back in the early '70s, McLean had a reputation of *not* being a place where smart Harvard Medical School students wanted to go for their psychiatric training. It was a second-rate place in terms of who was out there. The first-rate place was Mass Mental. McLean was kind of this aristocratic backwater where rich patients went. They got the second tier of the medical school people who either weren't very smart or weren't very broad. So I wasn't too interested in going there.

But I decided to interview, so I went out there, and Harvey was one of the two people who interviewed me. The other one was some aristocratic guy who saw on my resume that I had been a Rhodes scholar and started talking about Oxford. Harvey was this short, dark-haired, intense guy who sat behind a pile of books smoking a cigar. He did something no one else had done, he looked at my resume, closed the thing said, "Okay, we'll take you. What can I do to convince you to come here?"

Then we had a really wonderful conversation. I respected him because he was both an analyst and he was interested in the neurochemistry of psychiatric illness, which also interested me. He had a very kind, down to earth, modest, humble manner and it was on the basis of that, and seeing the beautiful grounds and tennis courts–I had been up to my elbows in the blood and gore of the inner city at the Beth Israel emergency room–that I said, "Hey, I'm coming."

That was in 1974, really the first year that some of the top guys at the medical school decided to come to McLean. A big reason for that was the new director, Shervert Frazier. He was a real hotshot. He had been president of the American Psychiatric Association, he was an eclectic psychiatrist, and he was hell-bent on making McLean into a good place. He was from Texas, and he spoke in this deep drawl, and would say things like, "Y'know, I'm going to get the best people here."

One of the best people in Frazier's stable was the forty-one-year-old Shein. The track is very fast at the Harvard Medical School, and Shein seemed to have covered more distance than any doctor of his generation. Shein hailed from a middle-class, not particularly religious family of reformed Jews living on the east side of Providence, Rhode Island, not far from Brown University. He attended Classical High School, the Providence equivalent of Boston's competitive Latin schools, and then went on to Cornell to study philosophy. His childhood friend John Livingstone, who later joined Harvey at Harvard Medical School and McLean, describes Shein as an intellectual plunger who would dive into huge bodies of art or knowledge–the works of Stravinsky or Wittgenstein—and emerge renewed and ready for cerebral combat. "He was an incredible thinker and conceptualist," says Livingstone. "He had an awesome, steel-trap mind. He was really argumentative, too. He'd argue with his parents, he would argue with me, he'd argue with anyone."

At Harvard, Shein landed a job in the virology lab of Dr. John Enders, a legendary figure in medical research who shared a 1954 Nobel Prize for his work on polio viruses. Later, he collaborated with Julius Axelrod, a biochemist who won the Nobel in 1970. One of Shein's analysts, Helen Tartakoff, wrote a famous paper about the "Nobel Prize complex" that affected extraordinarily precocious young men, and she noted that their addiction to ever-greater achievement and laurels could never be satisfied. Shein boasted to colleagues that he was the model for Tartakoff's maternally indulged, perennially disappointed superachiever.

In his mid-thirties, he reoriented his career to psychiatry and quickly made his mark at McLean. Before he turned forty, he was made director of residency training, the number-three clinical job at the hospital, and Frazier seemed to be grooming him for even more responsibility. In 1973, he appointed Shein psychiatrist-in-chief of Upham Hall, Louis Agassiz Shaw's old haunt, to add administrative experience to Shein's already impressive portfolio.

Starting in 1968, Shein had begun to publish research papers on suicide. Writing with his colleague Alan Stone, Shein asserted that psychiatrists and mental hospitals had to change the way they treated suicidal patients. Shein and Stone argued that most patients talk openly about their suicidal intentions and would be willing to discuss them with their therapists. But doctors too often were reluctant to place suicide front and center in the "therapeutic alliance," either because they feared upsetting an apparently stable patient or because they mistrusted their own motives. An over-concerned therapist might become enmeshed in a "rescue counter-transference," meaning that the therapist might fall victim to a fantasy that he or she could save the patient's life. The authors argued that suicide talk had to be brought into the open, not just in the doctor-patient relationship but throughout the hospital, to include nurses and ward aides in the course of treatment: "Suicidal intent must not be part of therapeutic confidentiality in a hospital setting."

Shein acknowledged that there are other possible avenues for treating suicide, for instance, electric shock. But if the therapist opts for the kind of open intervention that he and Stone espoused, one element is key:

> It is, of course, essential that the therapist take pains to make clear to the patient that he (the therapist) considers suicide to be a maladaptive action, irreversibly counter to the patient's sane interests and goals. . . . *It is equally essential that the therapist believe this;* if not, he should not be treating the patient within the delicate human framework of psychotherapy. [Emphasis added]

How odd. Why would Shein raise the possibility that a suicide counselor himself might not believe that life is worth living?

∽

The grim answer came in the summer of 1974. On the surface, Shein's life continued its upward trend. With his impressive achievements in neurovirology and in psychiatric research, he seemed to have a lock on tenure at Harvard. His last published paper was "Loneliness and Interpersonal Isolation: Focus for Therapy with Schizophrenic Patients." Shein no longer ran Upham, but he continued to oversee the residents and was handed some of the responsibilities of the clinical director, the hospital's second-in-command and chief flak-catcher. "He was being pushed to get more clinical experience so he could be clinical director," Irene Stiver said. "He was a brilliant researcher, but he was very young. I think he was overwhelmed." Shein was overloaded as usual, but he had been allowed to cut back on his psychiatric load to compensate. One of his few patients was Livingston Taylor, who had already launched a successful singing and songwriting career and who memorialized his therapist in his best-known song, "Carolina Day."

> *There were smoke, then booze, then tokes*
> *then Herc*
> *And my head were dead and gone*
> *And with Doctor Shein a lot of*
> *money and time*
> *And a few friends sticking around.*

One of Shein's friends from Upham, who remembers him cheerily navigating the character foibles of the assembled Mayflower screwballs, felt he looked sad now that he had moved "up the hill" into the administration building. "They were promoting him up on the hill, out of the valley [Upham], and nobody was really all that sure that he wanted to do it," this woman says. "He used to come back to Upham and visit. He was lonely, he talked longingly about the good old days. He seemed very stressed and not very happy. We all used to worry about him." A peer who was meeting Harvey for the first time immediately concluded that his colleague was experiencing an agitated depression: "His hands were shaking, he couldn't hold a pen." Although it was not widely known, Shein had switched away from his long-time analyst Tartakoff and had begun to see Dr. Elvin Semrad, a revered presence at Massachusetts Mental Health Center, who was sometimes regarded as a healer of last resort. "I remember joking with Harvey about the Harvard appointment," says Peter Choras, "and he told me, 'For the first time in my life, it looks like the road is going downhill, not uphill.' I assumed that he was thinking, 'It's easy now, I don't have to keep climbing.'"

On the evening of July 17, 1974, Shein invited the young residents from McLean to his home on Ward Street, in a comfortable neighborhood called Newton Centre. With the windows open to the still summer evening, Shein led a discussion of Sigmund

Freud's classic essay, "On Mourning and Melancholia." As he said farewell to his young guests, Shein told them he would be leaving on vacation the next day and would not see them for a while.

When Stephen Bergman walked into McLean the next day and began his usual bantering with the secretaries, they cut him short: "'Did you hear about Dr. Shein?' they asked, and I said no. 'He's dead. He killed himself last night.' And I said, 'Are you sure?' and they said, 'Oh yes,' and they knew how many pills he had taken, and what kind. I was totally stunned."

According to the police report, Shein had swallowed 500 milligrams of chloral hydrate, a common sleeping medication, which had been prescribed for his wife.* Mrs. Shein commented to one of the officers that her husband "had been depressed lately." The attending doctor at Newton-Wellesley Hospital failed to revive Shein, who had apparently taken the pills three hours before the ambulance arrived. Although the Newton police labeled the incident a suicide, the state medical examiner, Nathaniel Brackett Jr., was more circumspect. He noted that Shein died of "acute pulmonary edema assoc w therapeutic level of long acting barbiturate in the blood." He refused to speculate whether the death was a suicide or an accident. Harvey Shein, one of the most promising physicians of his generation, was dead at age forty-one.

∞

The death was shocking to Shein's numerous friends in and around McLean. Many found the institutional reaction horrifying. Just a day or two after Shein's suicide, the McLean psychiatrists gathered

---

*Five hundred milligrams of chloral hydrate is not a lethal dose, leaving open the possibility that the police report may be wrong or that Shein took the medication in a lethal combination with other drugs. The medical examiner noted the presence of a barbiturate in Shein's blood, but chloral hydrate is not a barbiturate.

in Conference Room A of the administration building for their regular Thursday meeting. The atmosphere was tense; Shein himself had presided over the previous week's meeting. Now, with one of their most cherished colleagues dead by his own hand, the assembled doctors were treated to a half-hour-long spiel on the trials and tribulations of the nursing department. "It was as if you were on the moon," remembers Dr. Richard Budson, then a brash young doctor with a reputation for confronting authority.

> We were sitting there all grief-stricken, and the nurses are giving their presentation. I just broke in and said, "I'm terribly sorry to interrupt the nursing department, but I think it's very important to process what happened to us." And for the next hour people shared their despair and dismay in a profound way, which had to happen.*

Peter Choras remembers,

> It was the worst-bungled way of managing it I had ever seen in my life, and not typical of Shervert Frazier at all. We got into a meeting a day or two after the suicide, and Sherv started to go through his agenda. It wasn't until one of the more prickly people at McLean, Dick Budson, said, "What are we doing here, Sherv? Harvey Shein is dead." There wouldn't have been any discussion unless Dick had broken into that. People were very protective of Sherv. . . . he was a lost man. Harvey was his heir apparent.

Shein's friends blamed Frazier for overloading Shein; "People were in a blaming mood," one psychiatrist remembers. Frazier contributed to the atmosphere of crisis and cover-up by refusing to acknowledge Shein's suicide. "Harvey M. Shein died suddenly

---

*Merton Kahne remembers walking ashen-faced into a similar meeting on November 22, 1963. The clinical director, Dr. Samuel Silverman, inquired what was wrong. "The president of the United States is dead," Kahne reported. "And they just went right on with the conference."

on July 18, 1974," was the official statement released over Frazier's signature. The newspaper obituaries reported that Shein had died of a heart attack, adding no further details. "Nobody would talk about it, but everybody knew," says Stiver. "People challenged Frazier at meetings I attended, and he would say, 'We don't know yet, we'll look into it, it's not at all certain. . . . ' And then he would close the conversation."

"Even though people knew that he had committed suicide, and they even knew what pills he had used," Stephen Bergman says,

the administration position was to deny that. . . . At one point, someone said to us residents—you've got to remember, these were my first two weeks as a psychiatrist—"No, no, that was just a rumor that he killed himself, he died of a fatal disease." That was the exact quote. I mean, wait a second! That was really, really, really destructive to us.

But the patients knew, lots of them. Imagine how the patients felt. He had been treating patients for depression, and here their doctor commits suicide!

John Livingstone recalls,

I remember being over at Harvey's house before the funeral, and Sherv was there, and this doctor from [the Psychoanalytic Institute] was there, and they were all taking over. The story was "death, cause unknown." There was the McLean brand name to protect, and of course the stigma to the Institute. It was damage control, spin doctoring. At that point, they were controlling what they could control.

Ever since he was involved in a plagiarism scandal in the 1980s, the once media-friendly Shervert Frazier has not been meeting with many journalists. But Frazier granted me an hour of his time—a fifty-minute-long psychiatric hour, because at age seventy-nine he was still seeing many patients—with no strings attached. He was as Bergman described him: intensely charming, intelligent, and above all, *Texan*—tall, gregarious, and outgoing—the kind of person one rarely encounters in the paneled halls of McLean Hospital. Among his other credentials, Frazier is the former Texas commissioner of mental health who cemented his academic reputation with an analysis of Charles Whitman, the deranged rifleman who killed sixteen students from his perch on the observation deck of the University of Texas Tower in 1966.

There is no question that one cannot ask a psychiatrist, and Frazier evinced no difficulty in talking about Harvey Shein. "He was admired and revered here," Frazier told me. "He was extremely bright, a good clinician and a good teacher." Shein's suicide

> had a great impact on me and on the staff. I was very sad. He was one of the brightest people I ever knew. I didn't know anything about what was going on in his mind, though I've learned a lot of it since—that he was in psychoanalysis, he was uncovering all kinds of things, that he was clinically depressed and that he had a couple of psychiatrists working with him and treating him.

How, I asked, did Shein die? At the time, Frazier replied, another doctor investigated Shein's death and concluded that it was accidental. "Now that I look back on it, I think maybe he had the feeling that because I was relatively new here, I didn't need to suffer the shock of suicide of a senior staff person. I think it was probably a suicide, if I had to add everything up that I've learned since."

Shein's colleagues traveled to Rhode Island to hear him eulogized at the Sugarman Funeral Home in Providence. "I went to his funeral, and I have never seen so many people crying in a funeral room in my life," remembers Dr. Edward Daniels. "The people I was sitting with didn't just sob, they were wailing." When discussing his friend's death, John Livingstone remembered Harvey's fascination with Wittgenstein and with Wittgenstein's contention that language could be a straitjacket that limited our ability to understand and describe the world. "Here's an example," Livingstone said to me:

Why did Harvey Shein commit suicide?

Well, we know the cause of his death; he killed himself because he swallowed an overdose. We can certainly come up with some reasons why he killed himself: He was overinvested in his career, he was losing ground in his personal relations. Or maybe it's a false question. Maybe it's not a question at all, but a statement of our own pain.

12

Life Goes On

The past twenty-five years have been a time of troubles for full-
service mental hospitals. The world has given up on long-term,
residential mental health care, or at least it has given up paying for
it. The moral therapy of Philippe Pinel and the twentieth-century
milieu therapy belong to history now. Insurance companies,
health maintenance organizations, and the federal government's
Medicare and Medicaid programs have been cutting back drasti-
cally on patient reimbursements for mental health. Psychopharmacology is the order of the day, and to health-care executives
that means quick diagnoses, rapid drug prescriptions, and hopes
for the best. Follow-up visits, generally limited to fifteen minutes,
are for discussing the drugs' side effects and altering the initial prescription. The new order is tough on patients and hard for psychiatrists too. "How can you know how somebody is doing if you
don't have enough time to ask, 'How are you feeling? How are
your relationships?'" asks Dr. Bruce Cohen, the current president
of McLean. Cohen, a molecular biologist by training, has devoted
his life to psychopharmacological research, but even he—as head

of the hospital, especially he—is uncomfortable with McMental health. "It is not enough to sit with somebody and say, 'So, do you have dry mouth? Have you had any hallucinations lately?' That doesn't work."

All over the country, hospitals like McLean have shut their doors. The Olmsted-designed Bloomingdale Asylum, like McLean, is trying to sell portions of its campus to developers to stay alive. During the writing of this book, Chestnut Lodge, Alfred Stanton's old stomping ground, went out of business. In the past quarter-century, McLean has had two near-death experiences, one in 1983, when the administration tried unsuccessfully to sell the hospital to a health-care conglomerate, and again in 1998, when Harvard considered closing it down. Although it is true that the hospital's most serious problems were economic, some of McLean's wounds were self-inflicted.

During the 1980s, McLean endured a series of embarrassing scandals. Three of its best-known doctors, including Edward Daniels, dubbed the "Mayor of McLean" for his legendary ability to keep his colleagues' psychiatric appointment books full, were accused of sexual harassment by female patients. The men all protested their innocence, but all relinquished their licenses to practice medicine. Then Shervert Frazier, the psychiatrist-in-chief and former head of the National Institute of Mental Health, lost his job in a plagiarism scandal that was reported on the front pages of both the *New York Times* and the *Boston Globe*. In the scheme of things, Frazier's infraction was relatively minor; his McLean colleagues felt he had been done in by jealous rivals on the Harvard campus. Once the brouhaha settled down, Frazier was quietly reinstated at McLean, although not in his former position. The publication of Stephen Bergman's roman à clef, *Mount Misery*, which depicted many of his former McLean colleagues as lunatic, sex-crazed pill-pushers, was an additional annoyance. The hospital's reputation within Boston's tight-knit medical community was badly tarnished.

But the news was not all bad. Frazier had raised money to build a new, modern, research building, and McLean doctors made discoveries of world-class significance. Dr. Seymour Kety published his famous "Danish twins" study that revealed an apparent genetic basis for schizophrenia, for which he won academic medicine's highest prize, the Albert Lasker Award. McLean doctors made important contributions to the development of Eli Lilly Company's "miracle pill," the antidepressant Prozac. Drs. Martin Teicher and Jonathan Cole published a controversial study warning of potential suicide risks among Prozac users, and Teicher became the lead scientist in an effort to reformulate the wonder drug. (That effort came to naught, and McLean lost several million dollars a year in anticipated royalties and license fees.) Throughout the decade, *U.S. News & World Report* continued to place McLean at or near the top of its list ranking the top private mental hospitals in the country.

Such successes made the bad economic news all the harder to swallow. The forty-day work-up of the Anne Sexton era was long gone. By the 1990s, insurance plans would generally pay for a thirteen-day stay at a mental hospital. Now the norm is five days. Alfred Stanton once diagnosed a patient by saying, "she has the eyes of a schizophrenic"; such intuitive, ludicrous diagnoses are a thing of the past. Psychiatrists and the insurance payers now hew closely to the syndromes and conditions described in the *Diagnostic and Statistical Manual of Mental Disorders-IV (DSM-IV)*, a detailed checklist of 297 mental diseases published by the American Psychiatric Association. (Homosexuality was included as recently as the *DSM-II* of 1974.) The *DSM* has attracted its share of ridicule—one writer noted that both President Bill Clinton and Hillary Rodham Clinton could be institutionalized under its conditions—but it is one of the few working documents recognized across the profession. Using the *DSM* and insurance-company guidelines, today's psychiatrist must stabilize, diagnose, treat—usually with a drug prescription—and release a disturbed man or woman in less than a week. Sometimes doctors carpet-bomb patients with prescriptions, hoping that one of the drugs will work. Here is a portion of a 1993 McLean medical record reproduced in *Under Observation,* an account by Dr. Alexander Vuckovic and Lisa Berger of a year on the McLean wards:

> On admission, she was taking Depakote 500 mg bid [twice daily], Trilafon 8 mg qhs [at bedtime], Zoloft 300 mg qAM [in the morning], Ativan 1 mg qid [once daily] prn [for] anxiety, Motrin 600 mg tid [three times daily] prn muscle pain, Firoicet 2 tabs bid prn H/A [headache], Spironolactone 25 mg qid prn premenstrual dysphoria, and Synthroid 0.2 mg as empirical mood stabilizer therapy.

By the early 1990s, explains Charles Baker, a former McLean board chairman, "we had an exquisite factory for a product we weren't selling anymore." Because private insurers were fleeing mental health, McLean started signing multimillion-dollar contracts with Medicare, which covers the elderly and the disabled, and with Medicaid, for lower-income patients. Doctors grumbled that McLean had become a "welfare hospital." If so, it was a money-losing welfare hospital. By the middle of the decade, McLean was losing up to $9 million a year, on an annual budget of only $80 million. The administration adopted desperate measures, laying off 30 percent of the staff. The hospital even sought the last refuge of the Brahmin dowager: They sold off the silver. In 1994, McLean put 238 separate items up for auction, including several lots of silver tea sets once used on the wards, a Paul Revere bowl, oriental rugs, some venerable grandfather clocks, dozens of pieces of hand-crafted furniture, and some paintings by American masters William Otis Bemis and John La Farge. Virtually all of the items had been languishing in the attics of Higginson House gathering dust. (Indeed, several rugs, tea sets, and pieces of furniture had already gone missing from the various halls, another powerful argument for the auction.) A hospital spokesman told the press that McLean hoped to net between $200,000 and $300,000 for the antiques. But many of the items had suffered damage from improper storage or had been overvalued by enthusiastic appraisers. In the end, McLean made only $160,000, one of many disappointments during this bleak period.

Morale at McLean was extremely low. Here is how one researcher who had been visiting the campus described the mood during the mid-1990s: Returning to McLean, she wrote,

> was a little like coming back to a tree-lined London neighborhood after the Blitz. . . . Administrators were frantically trying to cut costs. Nearly all the non-medical services—food preparation, laundry, lawn care—had been farmed out to independent contractors, and gardeners, cafeteria workers and others who had worked at the hospital, sometimes for decades, had been dismissed. Hospital units were opened and closed and reorganized like circus tents. . . . A third of the staff had been fired, the base salary of the rest would soon be cut in half, and many had left voluntarily in the hope that things would be better elsewhere. The administrators were behaving in ways that seemed sadistic to those under them, as if they were hoarding food in a severe famine. (However, they also probably saved the hospital from bankruptcy.) One clinician told me that at a rare meeting of clinicians, the hospital director showed a slide entitled "Your Options in Dealing With Managed Care" with a bulleted recommendation: "Move to Wyoming." No one laughed.

In 1997, Harvard consolidated all of its teaching hospitals into one huge company, Partners HealthCare System. For all the lip service accorded to the sanctity of the hospitals' medical mission, this was a garden-variety corporate merger. The managers at Partners had to demonstrate the efficiencies of the new combination, and eliminating overlapping services was an obvious first step. Partners had a small, top-notch psychiatry department at the downtown Massachusetts General Hospital and a money-losing, satellite operation sprawling over 240 acres of valuable real estate in Belmont. For the chairman of Partners, a former Harvard Business School dean, this was a no-brainer: Close down McLean.

Although no longer composed of Appletons, Lowells, and Putnams, McLean's board of trustees still included some the area's most influential businessmen and was not a group to be trifled with. They launched a furious counterattack. Pursuing a full-court diplomatic offensive with donors, academics, and state officials, the board succeeded in changing Partners's mind. To rescue the hospital, they devised the Hospital Re-Use Master Plan. McLean would sell off or give away 200 of its 250 acres and about half of its buildings, raising $40 million in the process. Olmsted's marvelous campus would be subdivided into luxury homes, an office park, and a housing complex for the elderly. The 300-bed hospital would become a 100-bed hospital. The trustees had destroyed a large portion of the hospital in order to save it.

∞

Years ago, when I described this project to a friend, he responded, "Oh, that sounds like a travel book." Working with McLean certainly felt like visiting a very foreign, very interesting country. I remember sitting with archivist Terry Bragg in his ground-floor office in the administration building when a young man dressed like a bicycle messenger—yellow nylon blouse, Spandex tights—walked through his open door. A delivery? No, the man had bicycled down to McLean from a campsite on Boston's North Shore, about thirty miles away. He had loaded his bike onto a train in South Carolina after seeing McLean's Dr. William Pollack on a public-television broadcast. Pollack was promoting his book *Real Boys*, about the challenges facing adolescent males, and he had struck a chord with this visitor. Pollack had an office across the hall, but he was not in. Terry gently told this man who had traveled a thousand miles to consult a doctor he had seen on television that Pollack might well show up later and that he was welcome to wait outside. The man walked back into the corridor, and Terry and I went back to work. "That happens all the time," he told me.

My McLean journey ended in President Bruce Cohen's spacious corner office, previously occupied by Franklin Wood, Alfred Stanton, and Shervert Frazier. The office is the closest thing the hospital has to a museum. The original Gilbert Stuart portrait of John McLean hangs above the fireplace. Among the antique gadgets on Cohen's shelf is a century-old microscope that belonged to August Hoch, one of the McLean doctors who traveled to Santa Barbara to care for International Harvester heir Stanley McCormick. While Cohen and I talked, sitting on opposite couches, I was gazing over his shoulder at a black marble bust of Rufus Wyman, the first superintendent of the Charlestown Asylum, who reported for work in 1818.

Bruce Cohen's job is, of course, light-years removed from that of Rufus Wyman. The first superintendent lived at the asylum and spent only five nights off the grounds in fourteen years. Cohen lives in Lexington with his wife and two children. He does resemble Wyman in that he takes hardly any vacation and never more than a week at a time. Wyman entertained patients at his dinner table and even threw rabbit shadows against the wall in the disturbed women's dormitory. Although Cohen has been around long enough to remember the discontinued Morning Reports, when McLean's ward chiefs would gather in the oak-paneled library across the hall to discuss "matters arising," he rarely visits the wards any more. Overseen by highly trained specialists in, say, geriatric psychiatry or pediatric psychopharmacology, McLean's different departments more or less run themselves.

Cohen is the very model of a modern mental health-care executive. He is, of course, a psychiatrist, and he is a prodigious researcher in his field of molecular biology. At age fifty-four, he has 307 scientific publications to his full or partial credit. No stranger to nerdspeak—he told me that his overlapping specialties of biochemical research and brain imaging "interdigitate quite well"—he is also an effective communicator and businessman who speaks the language of lucre. Cohen and his development officers raised more than $5 million from donors in 2000, a record amount and a significant contribution to the hospital's finances. He even has a sense of humor about McLean's financial predicaments, invoking the old business gag, "We're losing money on everything we do, but we'll make up for it in volume."

So what does Rufus Wyman's successor do? Like every hospital administrator in America, he frets about money and survival. The hospital loses money on teaching, on most research, and on all outpatient care. Patients who occupy beds are a break-even proposition, and patent royalties—a relatively new and important category—and donors' gifts help balance the books. But almost any line item in the budget can change quickly and unpredictably. During the 1997 passage of the Balanced Budget Act, McLean lost $2 million in Medicare reimbursements—poof!—two months before the beginning of its fiscal year. The prospective income stream from McLean's work on Prozac II likewise vanished when Eli Lilly's licensees abandoned the drug. Politicians and health maintenance organization executives now make the financial decisions that affect McLean's future; these men and women have become Bruce Cohen's core constituency. Cohen talks to them, lobbies them, jawbones them, and, in a not-so-subtle way, threatens them. The payers are always eager to take another bite out of McLean's hide, to cut back the minimum stays, or to slash the office visits from fifteen minutes to ten. And Cohen is willing to fight back. "I'm feeling a little combative," he said during our conversation.

It's time for us to be very frank and dig in our heels a little bit and tell people what it's costing us to provide this care. We're weaker, we're stigmatized compared with conventional medicine. People don't stand up and say, "I have bipolar disorder and I want you to pay for it!" Nonetheless, we have to say to some of the payers, "We just can't treat people for what you're paying us. Where is the breaking point in terms of changing these systems? How comfortable are you treating somebody in an unlocked setting, as opposed to a locked setting? In a day program as opposed to a residential program?"

Translation: We know who is disturbed and we know who is dangerously disturbed. Trust us to sort them out—and pay us to sort them out—or suffer the consequences.

It had not occurred to me that the $40 million Re-Use Master Plan would fail to save the hospital. I assumed the fresh capital would keep McLean alive for at least five years. But Cohen made no such assumptions. "Could the fate of an institution like this remain in the balance? Sure. Yes. I would be a fool to say to you that McLean's problems have been solved just because we look so much better now than we did five years ago." Cohen insists that he remains optimistic about McLean's future, but he knows the world of mental health funding is one where almost anything can go wrong and often does.

One small contributor to McLean's economic well-being is a brand-new ward called the Pavilion. For at least a decade, a small group of McLean doctors had been arguing for the creation of a high-end clinic to service the megarich, a sort of Mayo Clinic of mental health. The opportunity was there; the 1980s and 1990s produced their fair share of mixed-up plutocrats, and no one was competing for what Pavilion director Dr. Alexander Vuckovic calls "the old carriage-trade clientele." But appearances mattered. How could McLean beg Massachusetts for increased Medicaid funding or cry poor to the town of Belmont for tax relief if they were running an $1,800-a-day clinic for the Donald Trumps of the world? When McLean did finally open the Pavilion in 1998, they did not put out a press release; they still have not. I first learned about it when a patient friend of mine called to inform me that he had met his new wife in the most pleasant circumstances imaginable: recuperating at the Pavilion.

To be fair, McLean is not hiding its new gold-plated clinic under a bushel. The Pavilion advertises discreetly ("Unparalleled psychiatric evaluation and treatment. Unsurpassed discretion and service.") in upscale magazines. Furthermore, Vuckovic and his colleagues have talked up the Pavilion on the psychiatric grapevine. "McLean is still McLean," he says. "People in the profession know who we are. The name travels far."

Vuckovic, a psychopharmacologist by training, is smart and frothy, precisely the kind of person who should never be allowed to talk to journalists. When I entered his office at the Pavilion, he complained to me that he had spent part of the day arguing over a $25,000 bill with the Saudi Embassy. So much for "unsurpassed discretion." Of course, he was more than happy to show off his new ward, one of McLean's few unequivocal success stories in recent years.

The facility itself is unprepossessing, merely a group of renovated ground-floor suites on Wyman Hall. The Pavilion is the mental hospital equivalent of Club Med—one price, all included. For $1,800 a day, which is about double the price of a night on the regular wards, the patient receives virtually anything he or she wants: a psychiatric and psychopharmacological consultation, of course; a neurological evaluation; psychological testing; medical care; individual psychotherapy; and more. The bill is the bill; there are no separate, additional charges for pills, MRI scans, and the like. (The patient generally pays out of pocket.) The service has proved to be quite popular. When I went through in early 1999, all three suites were full, and McLean had a waiting list. Since then, three new suites have been added, and they, too, are fully occupied.

As in the old days, the Pavilion places much emphasis on "the little conveniences and luxuries of everyday life," to quote McLean's 1863 annual report. Pavilion residents enjoy better food than that served in the cafeteria, and they can request room service. Each suite has its own telephone, satellite television hookup, and private bathroom—amenities not found on the other wards. Fresh flowers appear every other day. The Pavilion is an un-locked ward, "for the less than super-crazy," as Vuckovic puts it. Like the Packard limousines of the Franklin Wood era, town cars whisk Pavilion patients to and from Boston and Cambridge. In-deed, the Pavilion is a lot like . . . the old McLean. Explains Peter Choras, one of the Pavilion's early promoters, "It's going back to what we used to do."

McLean is not the land of the cure. At the end of the day, the hospi-tal's goal is to succor patients, or right them, or just make them feel confident enough to give the real world, with all its ferocity and vicissitudes, one more try.

Returning to the hospital is a weighty issue for former patients. Rob Perkins talked with me about returning to Belmont, but it was not a high priority for either of us. Susanna Kaysen told me an old hall mate had once pressured her to return and had later committed suicide. It turned out that the woman was taking stock of her life before leaving it. When Kaysen's memoir, *Girl, Inter-rupted*, was published in 1993, a *Boston Globe* editor asked her to pose for a profile in front of South Belknap. She told him to go to hell. Kaysen has since returned on occasion, peddling her sar-donic celebrityhood. I once saw her amuse an appreciative audi-ence in McLean's modern cafeteria building with the line, "I'm always happy to be back at McLean . . . because it feels so great to *leave*." She did tell me that she enjoyed a visit with McLean's Manic-Depressive and Depressive Association during her book tour "because it was such a relief to be there, and to be under-stood. It was fun for them, and it was fun for me. They didn't ask, 'Are you still crazy?' It was like being with the native speakers of a language when you've been with non-native speakers, that's what I would liken it to."

The singing Taylors are often invited back, but James and Livingston do not like to go. McLean evokes no pleasant memories, and nobody presses the point. Their sister Kate, ebullient, beautiful, and gray-haired, has returned once. A few years ago, she traveled from Martha's Vineyard to Belmont to deliver the commencement address for the Arlington School, in Eliot Chapel. "I am happy to say that I am speaking to you as an alumna of the Arlington School," she told the boys and girls, and then she commented on her own life's journey:

> For some people life appears to proceed in a very predictable manner. Others of us sometimes find ourselves wondering what that must be like. Predictability does offer its share of comforts but at the same time it may also include its share of limitations.
>
> There are so many paths that you can now choose to set out upon in pursuing your personal quest. The scenery will certainly vary according to your particular choice. You needn't worry about getting to where you're going because, to paraphrase a line from songwriter Erica Wheeler, "You are the destination of your beautiful road."
>
> . . . By virtue of your presence here today, I am absolutely certain that you are uniquely qualified to pass on your legacy of kindness and compassion to others and that you will find your way to do it.
>
> It is your time, your turn to head out on that highway. Enjoy the twists and turns as well as the straightaway. Congratulations to you all and maybe I'll see you out there on that beautiful road.

Acknowledgments

This book could never have been written without the cooperation of two great Boston institutions, the *Boston Globe* and McLean Hospital.

The *Globe* allowed me ample time to pursue this project over the past several years. Editor Matt Storin and Managing Editor/Administration Louisa Williams approved my requests for leave. My supervisor, Deputy Managing Editor for Features Mary Jane Wilkinson, was extremely generous in granting me the flexibility I needed to finish this book. Living Section Editor Nick King sent me to Texas to write about the Anne Sexton poetry archive. Their successors, Mark Morrow and Fiona Luis, pretended not to notice when I sometimes seemed otherwise engaged. And I often relied on the excellent staff at the *Globe*'s library, overseen by Lisa Tuite, for research help.

McLean, led by Dr. Bruce Cohen, cooperated with me in every way that it could. The hospital's archivist and registrar, Terry Bragg, is an accomplished mental health historian who always made time for my inquiries. Audrey Martin, Terry's ever-present and helpful assistant, helped me in many ways. The hospital's librarian, Lyn Dietrich, chased down many an obscure journal article for me. My friend Roberta Shaw, the hospital's former director of public affairs, helped me arrange interviews, as did her successor, Cynthia Lepore. And special thanks for relaxing and informative conversation go to McLean's delightful "Mrs. B," Marion Bodeman.

I am grateful to these men and women for making themselves available for interviews: Dr. Abigail Stanton, Dr. Alfred Pope, Alice Brock, Dr.

Acknowledgments

Arthur Cain, Dr. Bernard Yudowitz, Mark Robart, Dr. Robert Coles, Dr. Bruce Cohen, Bruce Stanton, Bruce Cain, Dr. Richard Budson, Dr. Captane Thomson, Charles Baker, Clay Jackson, Constance Holian, Dr. David Lynn, Dr. Francis de Marneffe, Doug Drake, Douglas Holder, Dr. Edward Daniels, Eleanor Morris, Dr. Frederick Duhl, Dr. George Lawson, Golda Edinburg, Henry Langevin, Laurie Burgess, Barbara Schwartz, Parkman Shaw, the late Dr. Ruth Barnhouse, Frank Bidart, Susanna Kaysen, James Patterson, Dr. Paul Howard, Dr. Stephen Bergman, William Shine, Kate Taylor, James Taylor, Kenneth McElheny, Jack Thomas, Jeff Garland, Jim Garland, Dr. John Ellenberg, James Barr Ames, C. K. Williams, Dr. John Gunderson, Dr. John Livingstone, John Sheldon, Lloyd Schwartz, Jon Landau, Lois Ames, Robert Plunkett, Maria Pugatch, Michael James, Dr. Michael Sperber, Munson Hicks, Dr. Paul Dinsmore, Jonathan Bayliss, Paul Roberts, Rob Perkins, Dr. Peter Choras, Peter Storkerson, Dr. Phil Isenberg, Michael Punzak, Richard Wolfe, Dr. Shervert Frazier, Dr. Stephen Washburn, the late Irene Stiver, Dr. Thomas Bond, and Dr. Alexander Vuckovic. Some of these men and women were patients at McLean, and without their cooperation this book could not have been written. Several of my interview subjects asked to remain anonymous.

This book journey began at Stanford University, where I held a Knight Fellowship in journalism during the 1996/1997 academic year. Professor Diane Middlebrook encouraged me to pursue my book idea and introduced me to the writer Linda Gray Sexton, daughter of poet Anne Sexton. Linda jump-started my book by granting me access to the archives of her mother's McLean poetry seminar at the University of Texas's Harry Ransom Humanities Research Center. I had never worked in a university archive before, and the staff there—Cathy Henderson, Barbara Smith-LaBorde—and my landlady, the photographer Martha Campbell—made it a wonderful experience. Librarians and archivists are indeed the unacknowledged legislators of the universe, and I have many to thank: Karen Kukil, the curator of the Sylvia Plath Collection at Smith College; Stephen Jones and Diane Ducharme at Yale University's Beinecke Library; Lee Grady, Lisa Hinzman, and Geraldine Strey, who work with the McCormick Collection at the Wisconsin State Historical Society; Daniel Greenebaum, Rebecca Cape, and Saundra Taylor at Indiana University's Lilly Library; and Andrew Harrison at Johns Hopkins' Alan

Mason Chesney Medical Archives. I also received valuable research help from MIT's Liz Andrews, from Liz Locke, Charles Beveridge, Sylvia Nasar, Kathy McCabe, Dr. Richard Patterson, Richard Wolfe, Douglas Starr, Paul Alexander, Dr. Ronald Pies, Caroline Smedwig, Charles Mc-Laughlin, Sarah Payne Stuart, Betsy Lameyer, Hilda Golden, Elizabeth Padjen, Armond Fields, and Margery Resnick.

Every manuscript needs friends, and this one had many. Dr. Robert Coles, who interned at McLean, was an enthusiastic supporter and printed an excerpt in his magazine, *DoubleTake*. My friends David Warsh, Mark Feeney, and Joseph Finder never flagged in their enthusiasm for this project. Margo Howard provided some helpful contacts. Ellen Ratner became a key collaborator, as did Dr. Harold Williams. Dr. Merton Kahne, Paul Roazen, Peter Davison, Dr. Jeffrey Friedman, Terry Bragg, Mark Lee, and my wife Kirsten Lundberg all read portions of the manuscript and made important suggestions for improvement.

Geoffrey Shandler bought this book for PublicAffairs and kept his enthusiasm for the project even after he left the house. As a young student, PublicAffairs publisher and CEO Peter Osnos visited McLean with one of his professors and understands well Diane Middlebrook's observation that "McLean [has] always held an odd glamour as the hospital of choice for the occasionally mad artists of Boston." Lisa Kaufman did the actual work of editing the manuscript and hand-holding an occasionally tetchy author; she performed magnificently. My longtime friend and literary agent Michael Carlisle stayed with this project through thick and through thin.

To all: Thank you. And thank you to my family, Kirsten, Michael, Eric, and Christopher, because you are my wellspring of sanity and happiness.

Notes on Sources

EPIGRAPH

"Waking in the Blue" from *Selected Poems by Robert Lowell.* Copyright ©
1976 by Robert Lowell. Reprinted by permission of Farrar, Straus and
Giroux, LLC.

CHAPTER I
A VISIT TO THE MUSEUM OF THE CURES

The definitive source for accurate information on McLean history is Silvia Sutton's *Crossroads in Psychiatry: A History of the McLean Hospital,*
published in 1986 by the American Psychiatric Press. It is engagingly written and extremely informative. Sutton's research backstops much of my
writing about the early years of the hospital. I owe a great debt to Sutton's official history and to three general histories of psychiatry that I
consulted frequently: Edward Shorter's *A History of Psychiatry* (New
York: John Wiley and Sons, 1997); Albert Deutsch's *The Mentally Ill in
America* (New York: Columbia University Press, 1949); and *The History of
Psychiatry,* by Franz G. Alexander and Sheldon Selesnick (New York:
Harper and Row, 1966).

Rob Perkins's memoir is *Talking to Angels* (Boston: Beacon Press, 1996).
My information about the Taylor family comes from press clips (see the
Notes on Sources for Chapter 10) and my interviews. The primary ac-
counts of Robert Lowell's stays at McLean are the biographies by Ian

Hamilton (*Robert Lowell* [New York: Random House, 1982]) and Paul Mariani (*Lost Puritan* (New York: W.W. Norton and Co., 1994). Sylvia Nasar's biography of John Forbes Nash, *A Beautiful Mind* (New York: Simon and Schuster, 1998) has a chapter on his stay at McLean. Ray Charles discusses his arrest and experiences at McLean in his autobiography *Brother Ray* (New York: Dial Press, 1978). Copies of the Olmsted letters are in the McLean archives and are included in *The Papers of Frederick Law Olmsted* (Baltimore: Johns Hopkins University Press, 1981–1992). The famous quote ". . . confound them!" is to be found in Laura Wood Roper's biography *FLO* (Baltimore: Johns Hopkins University Press, 1973).

CHAPTER 2
BY THE BEST PEOPLE, FOR THE BEST PEOPLE

This chapter relies heavily on Sutton and on Nina Little's *Early Years of the McLean Hospital* (Boston: Francis A. Countway Library of Medicine, 1972). The William Folsom diaries appear in Little's book. Charles Beveridge and David Schuyler describe the Olmsted-Vaux asylum work in the introduction to *Creating Central Park*, volume 3 of *The Papers of Frederick Law Olmsted*.

CHAPTER 3
THE MAYFLOWER SCREWBALLS

The material on Emerson and on Jones Very comes from John McAleer's biography of Emerson (*Ralph Waldo Emerson: Days of Encounter* [Boston: Little, Brown, 1984]), which has a chapter on Very, and from Edwin Gittleman's biography of Very, *Jones Very: The Effective Years* (New York: Columbia University Press, 1967).

A family member shared John Warren's medical record with me. Douglas Starr published a fascinating account of the ether controversy in the *Boston Globe*, November 26, 2000. On this subject, I also consulted Richard Patterson's "Dr. Charles Thomas Jackson's Aphasia," *Journal of Medical Biography*, 1997. Details on the Hooper and Adams families are available in Otto Friedrich's *Clover* (New York: Simon and Schuster, 1979) and in Ernest Samuels's *Henry Adams* (Cambridge, Mass.: Belknap, 1989).

My account of William James's possible McLean sojourn derives from the cited interviews and from Linda Simon's *Genuine Reality: A Life of William James* (New York: Harcourt Brace and Co., 1998).

CHAPTER 4
THE COUNTRY CLUBBERS

Henry Hurd's article was published in the April 1898 issue of the *American Journal of Insanity;* Dr. Thomas Bond gave me his grandfather's unpublished memoir, "The Private World of McLean Hospital."

There is a very useful Stanley McCormick Archive at the State Historical Society of Wisconsin in Madison, containing many of his medical records. T.C. Boyle's novel *Riven Rock* (New York: Viking, 1998) is a fictionalized version of Stanley's plight. Armond Fields very generously shared his unpublished manuscript about Katharine McCormick, and MIT professor Margery Resnick also gave me her work on Katharine. Some McCormick family anecdotes come from Gilbert Harrison's *A Timeless Affair: The Life of Anita Blaine McCormick* (Chicago: University of Chicago Press, 1979), a biography of Stanley's philanthropically minded sister. The description of the art room and of "Julia Bowen's" life are in the McLean archives. The Myerson-Boyle paper is in the McLean archives. The daughter of "Priscilla Jenkins" shared her mother's McLean case file with me.

CHAPTER 5
THE SEARCH FOR THE CURE

A key text on this subject is Elliot Valenstein's 1986 book *Great and Desperate Cures* (New York: Basic Books). The description of Henry Cotton's work comes from the Edward Shorter history. The Talbott-Tillotson paper on hypothermia was published in the April 1941 issue of *Diseases of the Nervous System*. Freud's use of electroshock is reported in the Alexander and Selesnick history. "Total push" was described by Tillotson and Myerson in "Theory and Principles of the 'Total Push' Method in the Treatment of Chronic Schizophrenia," *American Journal of Psychiatry*, March 1931. Frank W. Kimball's "Hope for Tired Minds" appeared in the December 1946 and January 1947 issues of *Hygeia: The Health Magazine*.

Walter Freeman's hijinks are well documented in Valenstein. The complete history of lobotomies at McLean is Jack Pressman's *Last Resort: Psychosurgery and the Limits of Medicine* (Cambridge: Cambridge University Press, 1998).

CHAPTER 6
THE TALK CURE: FREUD AND MAN AT MCLEAN

Sutton discusses Boston's belated acceptance of Freud in her book. The story of James J. Putnam, Stanley Hall, and Freud's Clark University lectures is recounted in Paul Roazen's *Freud and His Followers* (New York: Knopf, 1975) and also in Ronald Clark's *Freud: The Man and the Cause* (New York: Random House, 1980).

There are two key sources for the tale of Dr. Horace Frink: Silas L. Warner's "Freud's Analysis of Horace Frink, M.D.: A Previously Unexplained Therapeutic Disaster," *Journal of the American Academy of Psychoanalysis,* 1994, and Lavinia Edmunds's "His Master's Choice," *Johns Hopkins Magazine,* April 1988. This article drew upon an archive donated to Johns Hopkins by Dr. Frink's daughter, Helen Frink Kraft, who confirmed a few details of her father's life in a letter to me.

The best short description of Scofield Thayer's life was written by Diane Ducharme, curator of Yale's *Dial*/Scofield Thayer Collection, and appears on the Beinecke Rare Book and Manuscript Library Web site (www.library.yale.edu.beinecke). Nicholas Joost's 1964 book *Scofield Thayer and the Dial* (Carbondale, Ill.: Southern Illinois University Press), is also a valuable source. All documents and correspondence quoted here are from the Yale collection.

Carl Liebman's story is recounted, anonymously, in Dr. David Lynn's "Freud's Analysis of A.B., a Psychotic Man, 1925–1930," *Journal of the American Academy of Psychoanalysis,* 1993. Most of the letters from Freud, Pfister, and others, first appeared in Dr. Lynn's article. McLean doctors shared portions of Liebman's record with me.

CHAPTER 7
WELCOME TO THE TWENTIETH CENTURY

As noted, Sutton's official history recounts the Tillotson-Salot story and also gives examples of Franklin Wood's parsimoniousness. On the personality of Dr. Alfred Stanton, my sources are his two surviving children and the many doctors quoted here who still remember him. Willis Bower's work is mentioned in Edward Shorter's history. Cristina Heilner granted me permission to quote from her brother's musical, *Close to Home*.

The suicide statistics come from Rose Coser's book *Training in Ambiguity* (New York: The Free Press, 1979) and also from "Some Notes on Thirty Years of Suicide at McLean Hospital," a paper presented at the hospital by Dr. George B. Lawson. Dr. Merton Kahne's analyses were published as "Suicides in Mental Hospitals: A Study of the Effects of Personnel and Patient Turnover," *Journal of Health and Social Behavior*, September 1968, and in "Suicide among Patients in Mental Hospitals: A Study of the Psychiatrists Who Conducted Their Psychotherapy," *Psychiatry*, February 1968.

The famous schizophrenia study undertaken by Dr. Alfred Stanton and Dr. John Gunderson, among others, was published as "Effects of Psychotherapy," *Schizophrenia Bulletin*, vol. 10, no. 4, 1984.

CHAPTER 8
THE MAD POETS' SOCIETY

Diane Wood Middlebrook's biography, *Anne Sexton* (Boston: Houghton Mifflin, 1991) is the definitive source for information on the poet. Sexton discussed her feelings about Sylvia Plath in "The Barfly Ought To Sing," an essay published in the fall 1966 edition of *TriQuarterly*.

Both the Hamilton and Mariani biographies describe Lowell's stays at McLean. The Sarah Cotting anecdote is in Sarah Payne Stuart's *My First Cousin Once Removed* (New York: HarperCollins, 1998). The Lowell letter to Elizabeth Bishop is from the Vassar College archive; the letter to Pound is from Yale's Beinecke Library. Both are reprinted by permission of the Estate of Robert Lowell.

Several books discuss Sylvia Plath, her mental illness, and her stay at McLean: Anne Stevenson's 1989 biography *Bitter Fame* (Boston: Houghton Mifflin), Paul Alexander's *Rough Magic* (New York: Viking Penguin, 1991), Peter Davison's *Half-Remembered: A Personal History* (New York: Harper and Row, 1973), Nancy H. Steiner's *A Closer Look at Ariel* (New York: Harper's Magazine Press, 1973), and Edward Butscher's *Sylvia*

Plath: Method and Madness (New York: Seabury Press, 1976). Quotes from Plath's journal can be found in *The Unabridged Journals of Sylvia Plath, 1950–1962*, edited by Karen Kukil (New York: Anchor Books, 2000). Ruth Barnhouse's letters are at the Sophia Smith Collection of Smith College and are used with permission.

The archive of the Anne Sexton poetry seminar is at the University of Texas's Harry Ransom Humanities Research Center, and her daughter and executor, Linda Gray Sexton, kindly granted me access to it. The Anne Sexton poetry fragment is quoted with Linda's permission. Robert Plunkett granted me permission to quote from his sister's poetry.

CHAPTER 9
STAYING ON: THE ELDERS FROM PLANET UPHAM

The details of Louis Shaw's life were pieced together from the interviews cited, from his Harvard reunion books, and from two memoirs: *The Day It Rained Fish,*" by Sidney Nichols Shurcliff (A.W. Shurcliff, 1991), and *Trooper: True Stories from a Proud Tradition,* by David Moran (Boston: Quinlan Press, 1986). Louis's lengthy and revealing will is on file in Essex County, Massachusetts.

McLean doctors shared details of the stories of the Ziegel brothers, Frank Everett, and Joan Wilkinson. Ray Charles's drug bust is described in his autobiography, in newspaper clips, and in Michael Lydon's *Ray Charles: Man and Music* (New York: Riverhead, 1998).

CHAPTER 10
DIAGNOSIS: "HIPPIEPHRENIA"

Dr. Alan Stone's comments on "hippiephrenia" appeared in the Summer 2000 issue of the *Boston Review.* In addition to the cited interviews, I also used the *Time* magazine cover story (March 1, 1971), a *New York Times Magazine* story (February 21, 1971), a long article by Timothy Crouse in *Rolling Stone* (February 18, 1971), and the *Rolling Stone* interview with James Taylor (September 6, 1979) to flesh out details of the Taylor family's pursuits in the early 1970s. The song fragment is quoted with James Taylor's permission.

Music therapist Paul Roberts shared his reports on his work at McLean with me.

CHAPTER 11
PHYSICIAN, HEAL THYSELF

Walter Jackson Freeman's book is *Psychiatrist: Personalities and Patterns* (New York: Grune and Stratton, 1968). The article by Charles Rich and Ferris Pitts appeared in the *Journal of Clinical Psychiatry* in August 1980. McLean doctors spoke to me about Doris Menzer-Benaron and Mark Altschule. There is a very interesting videotaped interview with Altschule in the Harvard Medical School's Countway Library of Medicine.

McLean provided me with Dr. Harvey Shein's curriculum vitae. Other biographical details came from interviews, primarily with his childhood friend John Livingstone. Shein and Stone published three major works on suicide: "Psychotherapy of the Hospitalized Suicidal Patient," *American Journal of Psychotherapy,* vol. 22: 15–25, 1968; "Psychotherapy Designed To Detect and Treat Suicidal Potential," *American Journal of Psychiatry,* March 1969; and "Monitoring and Treatment of Suicidal Potential within the Context of Psychotherapy," *Comprehensive Psychotherapy,* January 1969. Shein's paper on loneliness and isolation appeared in the *American Journal of Psychotherapy,* January 1974.

CHAPTER 12
LIFE GOES ON

There is no shortage of information on the parlous state of modern mental health. Two of my sources were Edward Shorter's history of psychiatry and T.M. Luhrmann's *Of Two Minds* (New York: Knopf, 2000), which provided the quote about McLean looking like London after the Blitz. *Under Observation,* by Dr. Alexander Vuckovic and Lisa Berger (New York: Ticknor and Fields, 1994), gives excellent insights into the workings of McLean during the early 1990s. The catalog for the art auction is in the McLean archives.

Index

Index

Dover, Thomas, 24
Dover's powder, 24
Dreams in the Mirror (Kennedy),
    102n
Drug therapy, 14, 24, 123–124, 124n.
    See also individual drugs
DSM-IV. *See Diagnostic and
    Statistical Manual of Mental
    Disorders-IV*
Dylan, Bob, 196–197

East House, 7, 166, 209, 212
ECT. *See* Electroconvulsive
    therapy
Edinburg, Golda, 143
*Effects of Psychotherapy in
    Schizophrenia, I and II*,
    139–141
Egasmoniz, António, 85–86, 217
Elders, the, 170
Electric light bath, 76
Electroconvulsive therapy (ECT),
    13, 13n, 81n, 155. *See also*
    Electroshock therapy
Electroshock therapy, 13, 78, 79,
    80, 81–83, 118, 123, 204, 221n
    and Plath, Sylvia, 154–155
    See also Electroconvulsive
    therapy
Eli Lilly Company, 235, 240
Eliot, George, 128
Eliot, T. S., 101
Eliot Chapel, 118, 135, 220, 244
Eliot family, 8
Ellenberg, John, 221–222
Ellis, George, 26
Emerson, Edward Bliss, 36

Emerson, Ralph Waldo, 35–36,
    37–38, 101, 161
Emerson, Robert Bulkeley, 35–36
"Encounter, Psychiatric Institute"
    (Plunkett), 163–164
Enders, John, 225
England, asylums in, 11
Epilepsy, 79n
Epsom salts, 24
Erikson, Erik, 45
Escapes, 212
Estelle's, 213
Ether, 38–39n
Etiquette, 26
Everett, Frank, 178–179, 187
Evipal, 75
Exploratory, insight-oriented
    (EIO) therapy, 140

Favill, Henry, 59
Fehmer and Page (architects), 50
Fever inducement, 74
Fitzgerald, F. Scott, 101
Fitzgerald, Zelda, 108–109
Fleury, Robert, 11
Fogg Museum, 182
Folsom, William, 26–30
Fomentation, 76
Food, at McLean Hospital, 28–29,
    64
Forced normalization theory,
    79n
"For the Union Dead" (Robert
    Lowell), 172
"Fragment for Anne" (Plunkett),
    164
France, asylums in, 10–11

PublicAffairs is a publishing house founded in 1997. It is a tribute to the standards, values, and flair of three persons who have served as mentors to countless reporters, writers, editors, and book people of all kinds, including me.

I.F. STONE, proprietor of *I. F. Stone's Weekly*, combined a commitment to the First Amendment with entrepreneurial zeal and reporting skill and became one of the great independent journalists in American history. At the age of eighty, Izzy published *The Trial of Socrates*, which was a national bestseller. He wrote the book after he taught himself ancient Greek.

BENJAMIN C. BRADLEE was for nearly thirty years the charismatic editorial leader of *The Washington Post*. It was Ben who gave the *Post* the range and courage to pursue such historic issues as Watergate. He supported his reporters with a tenacity that made them fearless and it is no accident that so many became authors of influential, best-selling books.

ROBERT L. BERNSTEIN, the chief executive of Random House for more than a quarter century, guided one of the nation's premier publishing houses. Bob was personally responsible for many books of political dissent and argument that challenged tyranny around the globe. He is also the founder and longtime chair of Human Rights Watch, one of the most respected human rights organizations in the world.

For fifty years, the banner of Public Affairs Press was carried by its owner Morris B. Schnapper, who published Gandhi, Nasser, Toynbee, Truman, and about 1,500 other authors. In 1983, Schnapper was described by *The Washington Post* as "a redoubtable gadfly." His legacy will endure in the books to come.

Peter Osnos, *Founder and Editor-at-Large*

Made in the USA
Lexington, KY
31 March 2010